THE EASIEST DASH DIET COOKBOOK FOR BEGINNERS

INCREASE ENERGY LEVELS
AND LOWER BLOOD PRESSURE NATURALLY

Table Of Contents

CHAPTER 5: LUNCH

CHAPTER 6: DINNER

CHAPTER 7: SIDES

CHAPTER 8: VEGETABLES

CHAPTER 9: EGGS AND DAIRY RECIPES

Introduction

The DASH Diet is a diet used to lower blood pressure. It is also known as DASH (Dietary Approaches to Stop Hypertension). This diet is primarily used to treat people with high blood pressure, but has also been shown to be effective for certain complications of diabetes, and may also reduce the risk of heart disease.

The DASH diet encourages the consumption of nutrient-rich foods that are also lower in energy. When following this diet, 2,000 calories a day assume the use of a food totaling system.

This diet, due to its low content of saturated fat and its high content of fruit and vegetables, promotes the reduction of heart disease. It can be especially helpful for controlling the amount of sodium consumed per day, and reducing the risk of strokes and high blood pressure.

The guidelines of DASH are mainly aimed at reducing the amount of salt consumed. In fact, salt is eliminated as completely as possible or at least reduced. There is a limited number of low-fat products, white bread and rice that can be consumed.

It is not only the salt, but also the fat consumption that is limited on this diet. It is primarily aimed at reducing blood pressure and cholesterol. It was introduced in 1993 by the National Heart, Lung, and Blood Institute.

The diet is not designed to be followed as long as the others. It is a diet to think of as a solution to a possible dietary problem in the long term and therefore for a limited period of time. There is no fixed period for which this diet is to be followed.

In general, the DASH diet provides for a lower amount of salt, saturated fat, and cholesterol in the body. This is achieved by a lowering of blood pressure and by a regulation of the other substances. It is also necessary to have the approval of the physician.

This diet is very low in sodium and permits a moderate amount of potassium. The food is primarily based on vegetable or low-density fruits and grains, cereals, poultry and fish. There is a reduction in sodium and carbohydrates which are rich in vitamins and minerals, sweets and alcohol, white bread and rice, and dairy products.

Dash Diet has gained popularity in the past few years as it is extremely helpful in strengthening metabolism and controlling hypertension. Contrary to the popular belief that while following the dash diet, one gets to only eat vegetarian foods while you get a balanced diet that includes fresh fruits, vegetables, nuts, low-fat dairy products and whole grains. You do not have to completely cut down on meat; instead you just have to reduce sodium and fat content from your everyday diet.

The diet also has many health benefits as it helps in reducing hypertension and obesity lowering osteoporosis and preventing cancer. This well-balanced diet strengthens metabolism which further helps in decomposing the fat deposits stored in the body. This, in turn, enhances the general health of a person.

This diet is easy to follow as you get to everything but in a healthier fashion and limited quantity.

Talking about the DASH diet outside the theory and more in practice reveals more of its efficiency as a diet. Besides excess research and experiments, the true reasons for people looking into this diet are its certain features. It gives the feeling of ease and convenience, which makes the users more comfortable with its rules and regulations.

The DASH diet is very disciplined and that is its main problem. It needs a serious commitment on the part of the person who decides to use it. This diet is not recommended for everyone. The persons who are older, have diabetes, have diseases of the heart, or are currently on medication that has anticoagulants should not use the diet. For the reason that the diet requires them to gradually reduce the levels of ascorbic acid found in the body and the amount of salt consumed, not to mention if the medications are in fact anticoagulant.

CHAPTER 1:

What Is the DASH Diet?

Endorsed by the United States National Heart, Lung, and Blood Institute, the DASH (Dietary Approaches to Stop Hypertension) diet studies the nutrient composition of food items to prepare unique dietary strategies that help to reduce high blood pressure. The diet is a result of the engineering done by bio-scientists and lawmakers to find the components that must be eliminated from one's diet to control the rise of blood pressure.

The DASH diet came about because the number of people complaining of high blood pressure almost doubled in the last two decades. This led medical experts, along with the United States Department of Health and Human Services, to find ways to deal with hypertension and eliminate the various risks that are associated with high blood pressure. After a careful study, the researchers found that people who prefer to consume more vegetables or who followed a plant-based diet showed fewer signs and cases of rising blood pressure. This, therefore, became the foundation of the DASH diet.

In the DASH diet, the person focuses on consuming foods that are non-processed and more organic. Whole grains, fruits, vegetables, and lean meats form the essential components of this diet technique. In extreme cases, the person showing major signs of heart-related ailments due to high blood pressure is also advised to go vegan for some time to lower issues related to hypertension.

The diet also follows a strict method of using salt. Because too much salt and oil significantly raise the blood pressure in the human body, the dietary guidelines of the DASH diet significantly reduce the intake of salt. The recipes in the DASH diet are a wholesome mix of green vegetables, natural fruits, low-fat dairy foods, and lean protein such as chicken, fish, and a lot of beans. Besides limiting the intake of salt, the rule of thumb is to minimize food items rich in red meat, processed sugars, and composite fat.

As per the standard practice, anyone following the DASH diet is advised not to consume more than one teaspoon (2,300 mg) of sodium in a day.

The diet is safe to follow and is also accredited by the United States Department of Agriculture (USDA). The US Dietary Guidelines also included the DASH diet as one of three healthy diets recommended in 2015-2020.

Benefits of the DASH diet

The benefits of the DASH diet go beyond reducing hypertension and heart ailments.

Controlling blood pressure: The force exerted on our blood vessels and organs when the blood passes through them is a measure of blood pressure in the human body. When blood pressure increases beyond a certain level, it can lead to various bodily malfunctions, including heart failure.

Blood pressure is counted in two numbers: systolic pressure (pressure exerted in the blood vessels when the heart beats) and diastolic pressure (pressure exerted in the blood vessels when the heart is at rest). The normal blood systolic pressure in adults is below 120 mmHg, while the diastolic pressure is typically below 80 mmHg. Anyone over these limits is said to be suffering from high blood pressure.

The restriction of sodium intake and reliance on vegetables, healthy fat, lean meat, and fruits in the DASH diet greatly controls blood pressure. In fact, the lower one's salt intake, the lower one's blood pressure. Effective use of the DASH diet can control the systolic blood pressure by an average change of 12 mmHg and can control the diastolic blood pressure by 5 mmHg.

The DASH diet is not reserved for people suffering from hypertension; it can also work well for people with normal blood pressure. The trick is to consume normal amounts of salt along with the dietary recommendations given in the DASH diet.

Weight loss: People with high blood pressure are advised to maintain their weight, as extra weight may translate into health complications. Obesity along with high blood pressure can lead to heart and organ failure. With the help of the DASH diet, one can lower their blood pressure while also lowering their weight. The credit for this goes to the healthy foods recommended in the DASH diet. The person is advised to cut down on their daily calorie count to lose weight.

Further, the DASH diet has shown signs of other health benefits:

Fights cancer risk: People on the DASH diet have a lower risk of colorectal and breast cancers.

Checks metabolic syndrome: The diet reduces the risk of metabolic syndrome.

Controls diabetes: The diet is very beneficial for people with type 2 diabetes.
Heart diseases: The diet reduces the risk of heart disease and stroke.

CHAPTER 2:

What to Eat and Avoid on Dash Diet

Grain Products

What to eat	Eat occasionally	What to avoid
Brown rice Whole-grain breakfast cereals Bulgur Quinoa Oatmeal Popcorn Rice cakes	Whole-wheat pasta Whole-wheat noodles	White rice Regular pasta White bread

Use only whole grains because they are richer in fiber and nutrients. They are low-fat and can easily substitute butter, cheese, and cream.

Vegetables

What to eat	What to avoid
All fresh vegetables and greens Low-sodium canned vegetables	Regular canned vegetables

Vegetables are the richest source of fiber, vitamins, potassium, and magnesium. You can use vegetables not only as a side dish but also as a topping, spread, or meat-free main dish substitutes.

Fruits and Berries

Fruits and berries have the same vital benefits as vegetables. They are rich in minerals and vitamins.

One more advantage of fruits and berries is their low-fat content. They can be a good substitution for desserts and snacks. Fruit peels contain the highest amount of fiber and useful nutrients in comparison with fruit flesh.

What to eat	Eat occasionally	What to avoid

All fruits and berries (pineapple, apple, mango, pears, strawberries, raspberries, dates, apricots, etc.)	Grapefruit Orange Lemon	Sugar added canned fruits Coconut

Dairy

Dairy products are the main source of D vitamins and calcium. The only restriction for dash diet followers is saturated and high-fat dairy products.

Note: you can substitute dairy products with nut, almond, cashew, and soy milk.

What to eat	Eat occasionally	What to avoid
Low-fat or fat-free cheese Low-fat or fat-free yogurt Low-fat or fat-free milk/percent milk Low-fat or fat-free skim milk Low-fat or fat-free frozen yogurt	Low-fat cream Low-fat buttermilk	Full-fat cream Full-fat milk Full-fat cheese Full-fat yogurt

Meat and Poultry

Meat is rich in zinc, B vitamins, protein, and iron. There is a wide variety of recipes that will help you to cook meat in different ways. You can broil, grill, bake or roast it but anyways it will be delicious.

Note: avoid to eat skin and fat from poultry and meat.

What to eat	Eat occasionally	What to avoid
Skinless chicken breast Skinless chicken thighs Skinless chicken wings Skinless drumsticks Chicken fillet	Lean cuts of red meat (pork, beef, veal, lamb) Eggs	Fat cuts of meat Pork belly Bacon Fat

Fish and Seafood

The main benefits you will get from the fish which is high in omega-3 fatty acids. All types of seafood and fish are allowed on the dash diet. You will find the best fish choice for the dash diet below.

What to eat	What to avoid
Salmon	High sodium canned fish and

Herring Tuna	seafood

Nuts, Seeds, and Legumes

This type of product is rich in fiber, phytochemicals, potassium, magnesium, and proteins. It has the ability to fight cancer and cardiovascular disease.

Nuts, seeds, and legumes are high in calories and should be eaten in moderation. Add them into your salads or main dishes, they will saturate the taste.

What to eat
All types of seeds
All types of nuts
All types of legumes

Fats and Oils

The main function of fats is to help in absorbing vitamins; nevertheless, the high amount of fats can lead to developing heart diseases, obesity, and diabetes.

According to the dash diet, your daily meal plan shouldn't include more than 30% of fats of daily calories.

What to eat	Eat occasionally	What to avoid
Margarine Vegetable oils	Low-fat mayonnaise Light-salad dressings	Butter Lard Solid shortening Palm oil

Sweets

It is not necessary to cross out all sweets from your daily diet but it is important to follow some restrictions that the dash diet provides: choose sugar-free, low-fat/fat-free sweets or replace them with fruits and berries.

What to eat	Eat occasionally	What to avoid
Fruit/berries sorbets Fruit ice Graham crackers Honey Sugar-free fruit jelly	Hard candy Splenda Aspartame (NutraSweet, Equal) Agave syrup Maple syrup	Biscuits Crackers Cookies Soda Unrefined sugar Table sugar Sweet junk food

Alcohol and Caffeine
You should limit alcohol to 2 drinks per day for men and up to 1 or fewer drinks for women.
Note: alcohol and caffeine consumption can be forbidden totally if it is required according to a medical examination.

CHAPTER 3:

Tips for DASH Diet Success

Make a list before going to the store. Often, we don't plan before going to the grocery store. This can result in buying more food than you needed and getting distracted by non-healthy foods that aren't right for the DASH diet. Find healthy and delicious DASH diet recipes beforehand and write down all the ingredients you need. You won't be tempted by the other food in the grocery store because your mind will be set on the delicious meals you've already thought of that are in agreement with the DASH diet rules.

Eat before going shopping. Similar to the last tip, never shop hungry. When you're hungry you have a wandering eye that will want to eat more than what's on your list. Also, when you're hungry you may gravitate towards snacks and processed foods for a quick fix to your hunger. Processed foods are a big no for the DASH diet since they're often high in sodium, so avoid the temptations by not shopping when you're hungry.

Keep DASH-approved food at home. Diets are all about avoiding temptation. When you keep junk food and sweets around next to your healthy options, you're more likely to pick the former. However, if you have the basic DASH food staples, like grains, vegetables, nuts, and fruit you're more likely to eat these out of convenience, rather than leave to go to the store and indulge in junk food. Out of sight, out of mind.

Cook's wear is important to consider. Certain tools in the kitchen will be more beneficial to the DASH diet than others. Here are three kitchen cook wear items that you should have in your kitchen. The first is a nonstick pan. This eliminated the need to coat the pan with oil or butter. Since oils and fats are low on the list of food groups you should be eating, it's best to cut down on these fats when you can. Next, a steamer. Steamers are great because all it adds to your DASH-approved vegetable is water. Healthy food is cooked to perfection. Lastly, a spice mill to grind up whole, natural spices so you avoid livening up your meals with salt.

Rinse off canned foods. Canned vegetables are a quick way to buy vegetables, prepare them, and have them last. They're perfectly okay to eat under the DASH diet. However, the juice in the can carries a lot of excess salt. Get rid of most of this excess by simply rinsing your vegetables off with water before you eat them.

Don't be afraid to ask. It can feel difficult to go out to eat and still maintain your diet. If you want to order something off the menu but are afraid that the salt content may be too high, ask the waiter to ask the chef. Many people have dietary restrictions and you're not a burden for asking. This way, you can eat guilt-free and enjoy your meal. Also, check the ingredients. If the menu doesn't list all of the ingredients on the page, ask your waiter. They may have to ask the chef or sometimes a deeper nutritional value of each item is available on the restaurant's website.

Drink only water. This is a hard feat for some and an easy one for others. If you're a big soda or juice fan, this tip is for you. Sugars, even "fake sugars" like Splenda are put into common prepackaged drinks. Even when buying juice, you may think it'll be fine because it's a serving of your fruit intake for the day. This may be true, however there may also be so many added sugars to the drink that the one fruit serving was ultimately canceled out by the influx of sugar in the juice. You can even branch out to sparkling water or tea but steer clear of drinks with hidden sugars.

Ask for the lunch portion. It's important with the DASH diet to keep your calories at the respected amount. Often at restaurants, a large portion is given and when it's on your plate, your mind feels obligated to eat it. Ask for the lunch portion if you're out to dinner and have them put the rest in a to-go box. Not only are you sticking with your diet this way, but you also are saving money with an extra portion for later.

Fruit for dessert. This tip works both at home and in restaurants. If you're craving something sweet to finish off your meal, turn to dessert. If regular fruit doesn't satisfy you, there are tons of recipes on how to turn an average dish of fruit into a yummy dessert and still maintain the health that the fruit on its own originally had. If at a restaurant, go for a fruit sorbet or parfait. It may have some sugars, but much less than a devil's food cake would. You'll be sticking to the DASH diet while enjoying something sweet.

Cut back on meat. This can be a fast or gradual process, depending on how big of a meat eater you are. Much of the sodium we try to avoid comes from meat. You don't have to cut out all meat from the jump but reduce your intake. If you eat meat every day, try eating only 6 days a week. The same can be applied to meals, if you eat meat at every meal, take it down to only 2 meals. You can even just reduce your serving size of meat that you eat at each meal.

CHAPTER 4:

Breakfast

Shrimp Skillet

Preparation time: 10 minutes
Cooking time: 25 minutes
Servings: 5
Ingredients:

- 2 bell peppers
- 1 red onion
- 1-pound shrimps, peeled
- ½ teaspoon ground coriander
- ½ teaspoon white pepper
- ½ teaspoon paprika
- 1 tablespoon butter

Directions:

1. Remove the seeds from the bell peppers and cut the vegetable into the wedges.
2. Then place them in the skillet.
3. Add peeled shrimps, white pepper, paprika, and butter.
4. Peel and slice the red onion. Add it in the skillet too.
5. Preheat the oven to 365f.
6. Cover the skillet with foil and secure the edges.
7. Transfer it in the preheated oven and cook for 20 minutes.
8. When the time is over, discard the foil and cook the dish for 5 minutes more -use ventilation mode if you have.

Nutrition: calories 153, fat 4, fiber 1.3, carbs 7.3, protein 21.5

Coconut Yogurt with Chia Seeds

Preparation time: 2 hours

Cooking time: 10 minutes

Servings: 4

Ingredients:

- 1 probiotic capsule -yogurt capsule
- 1 cup of coconut milk
- 1 tablespoon coconut meat
- 4 tablespoons chia seeds

Directions:

1. Pour coconut milk in the saucepan and preheat it till 108F.
2. Then add a probiotic capsule and stir well. Close the lid and leave the coconut milk for 40 minutes.
3. Meanwhile, shred coconut meat.
4. When the time is over, transfer the almond milk mixture into the cheesecloth and squeeze it. Leave it like this for 40 minutes more or until the liquid from yogurt is squeezed.
5. After this, transfer the yogurt into the serving glasses.
6. Add chia seeds and coconut meat in every glass and mix up well.
7. Let the cooked yogurt rest for 10 minutes before serving.

Nutrition: calories 177, fat 16.9, fiber 3.9, carbs 6.5, protein 2.6

Chia Pudding

Preparation time: 15 minutes
Cooking time: 3 minutes
Servings: 4
Ingredients:

- 2 cups almond milk
- 8 tablespoons chia seeds
- 1 oz blackberries
- 1 tablespoon Erythritol

Directions:

1. Preheat almond milk for 3 minutes, then remove it from the heat and add chia seeds.
2. Stir gently and add Erythritol. Mix it up.
3. In the bottom of serving glasses put blackberries.
4. Then pour almond milk mixture over berries. Let the pudding rest for at least 10 minutes before serving.

Nutrition: calories 331, fat 31.9, fiber 6.7, carbs 11.8, protein 4.6

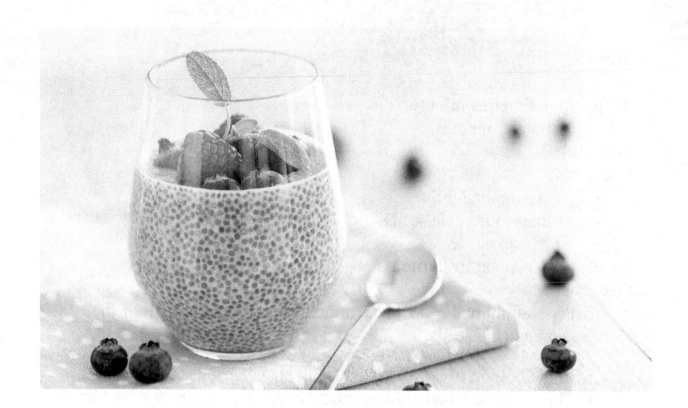

Egg Fat Bombs [1]

Preparation time: 10 minutes
Cooking time: 10 minutes
Servings: 4

Ingredients:

- 4 oz bacon, sliced
- 4 eggs, boiled
- 1 tablespoon butter, softened
- ½ teaspoon salt
- ½ teaspoon ground black pepper
- 1 tablespoon mayonnaise

Directions:

1. Line the tray with the baking paper. Place the bacon on the paper.
2. Preheat the oven to 365F and put the tray inside.
3. Cook the bacon for 10 minutes or until it is light brown.
4. Meanwhile, peeled and chop the boiled eggs and transfer them in the mixing bowl.
5. Add ground black pepper, mayonnaise, and salt.
6. When the bacon is cooked, chill it little and finely chop.
7. Add bacon in the egg mixture. Stir it well.
8. Add softened butter and mix up it again. With the help of the scoop make medium size balls. Before serving, place them in the fridge for 10 minutes.

Nutrition: calories 255, fat 20.3, fiber 0.1, carbs 1.2, protein 16.1

Morning "Grits"

Preparation time: 10 minutes
Cooking time: 10 minutes
Servings: 4

Ingredients:

- 1 ½ cup almond milk
- 1 cup heavy cream, whipped
- 4 tablespoon chia seeds
- 3 oz Parmesan, grated
- ½ teaspoon chili flakes
- ½ teaspoon salt
- 1 tablespoon butter

Directions:

1. Pour almond milk in the saucepan and bring it to boil.
2. Meanwhile, grind the chia seeds with the help of the coffee grinder.
3. Remove the almond milk from the heat and add grinded chia seeds.
4. Add whipped cream, chili flakes, and salt. Stir it well and leave for 5 minutes.
5. After this, add butter and grated parmesan. Stir well and preheat it over the low heat until the cheese is melted.
6. Stir it again and transfer in the serving bowls.

Nutrition: calories 439, fat 42.2, fiber 4.4, carbs 9.6, protein 10.7

Scotch Eggs

Preparation time: 15 minutes
Cooking time: 15 minutes
Servings: 4
Ingredients:
- 4 eggs, boiled
- 1 ½ cup ground beef
- 1 tablespoon onion, grated
- ½ teaspoon ground black pepper
- ½ teaspoon salt
- ½ teaspoon dried oregano
- ½ teaspoon dried basil
- 1 tablespoon butter
- ¾ cup of water

Directions:
1. In the mixing bowl, mix up together ground beef, grated onion, ground black pepper, salt, dried oregano, and basil.
2. Peel the boiled eggs.
3. Make 4 balls from the ground beef mixture. Put peeled eggs inside every ground beef ball and press them gently to get the shape of eggs.
4. Spread the tray with the butter and place ground beef eggs on it.
5. Add water.
6. Preheat oven to 365F and transfer the tray inside.
7. Cook the dish for 15 minutes or until each side of Scotch eggs is light brown.

Nutrition: calories 188, fat 13.4, fiber 0.2, carbs 0.9, protein 15.4

Bacon Sandwich

Preparation time: 15 minutes
Cooking time: 20 minutes
Servings: 2
Ingredients:

- 1 oz bacon, sliced -4 slices
- 4 eggs, separated
- 2 teaspoons ricotta cheese
- ¾ teaspoon cream of tartar
- 1 teaspoon flax meal, ground
- 2 lettuce leaves

Directions:

1. Whisk the eggs yolks with 1 teaspoon of ricotta cheese until you get a soft and light fluffy mixture.
2. After this, whip together egg whites with remaining ricotta cheese, salt, and cream of tartar. When the mixture is fluffy, add ground flax meal and stir gently.
3. Preheat the oven to 310F.
4. Gently combine together egg yolk mixture and egg white mixture.
5. Line the tray with baking paper.
6. Make the 4 medium size clouds from the egg mixture using the spoon.
7. Transfer the tray in the oven and cook them for 20 minutes or until they are light brown.
8. Meanwhile, place bacon slices in the skillet and roast them for 1 minute from each side over the medium-high heat.
9. Chill the bacon little.
10. Transfer the cooked and chilled egg clouds on the plate.
11. Place bacon onto 2 clouds and then add lettuce leaves. Cover them with the remaining egg clouds.
12. Secure the sandwiches with toothpicks and transfer in the serving plate.

Nutrition: calories 218, fat 15.5, fiber 0.4, carbs 2.3, protein 17.2

Noatmeal

Preparation time: 10 minutes
Cooking time: 10 minutes
Servings: 3
Ingredients:

- 1 cup organic almond milk
- 2 tablespoons hemp seeds
- 1 tablespoon chia seeds, dried
- 1 tablespoon Erythritol
- 1 tablespoon almond flakes
- 2 tablespoons coconut flour
- 1 tablespoon flax meal
- 1 tablespoon walnuts, chopped
- ½ teaspoon vanilla extract
- ¼ teaspoon ground cinnamon

Directions:

1. Put all the ingredients except vanilla extract in the saucepan and stir gently.
2. Cook the mixture on the low heat for 10 minutes. Stir it constantly.
3. When the mixture starts to be thick, add vanilla extract. Mix it up.
4. Remove the noatmeal from the heat and let it rest little.

Nutrition: calories 350, fat 30.4, fiber 8.4, carbs 16.9, protein 9.1

Breakfast Bake with Meat

Preparation time: 10 minutes
Cooking time: 30 minutes
Servings: 4

Ingredients:

- 1 cup ground beef
- 1 cup cauliflower, shredded
- ½ cup coconut cream
- 1 onion, diced
- 1 teaspoon butter
- ½ teaspoon salt
- ½ teaspoon paprika
- ½ teaspoon garam masala
- 1 tablespoon fresh cilantro, chopped
- 1 oz celery root, grated
- 1 oz Cheddar cheese, grated

Directions:

1. Mix up together garam masala mixture, celery root, paprika, salt, and ground beef.
2. Mix up together shredded cauliflower and salt.
3. Spread the casserole tray with butter.
4. Make the layer of the ground beef mixture inside the casserole tray.
5. Then place the layer of the cauliflower mixture and diced onion.
6. Sprinkle it with grated cheese and fresh cilantro, Add coconut cream.
7. Cover the surface of the casserole with the foil and secure the lids.
8. Preheat the oven to 365F.
9. Place the casserole tray in the oven and cook it for 30 minutes.
10. When the time is over, transfer the casserole from the oven, remove the foil and let it chill for 15 minutes.
11. Cut it into the serving and transfer in the serving bowls.

Nutrition: calories 192, fat 14.7, fiber 2.1, carbs 6.5, protein 10

Breakfast Bagel

Preparation time: 15 minutes
Cooking time: 30 minutes
Servings: 3
Ingredients:
- ½ cup almond flour
- 1 ½ teaspoon xanthan gum
- 1 egg, beaten
- 3 oz Parmesan, grated
- ½ teaspoon cumin seeds
- 1 teaspoon cream cheese
- 1 teaspoon butter, melted

Directions:
1. In the mixing bowl, mix up together almond flour, xanthan gum, and egg.
2. Stir it until homogenous.
3. Put the cheese in the separate bowl, add cream cheese.
4. Microwave the mixture until it is melted. Stir it well.
5. Combine together cheese mixture and almond flour mixture and knead the dough.
6. Roll the dough into the log.
7. Cut the log into 3 pieces and make bagels. Line the tray with baking paper and place bagels on it.
8. Brush the meal with melted butter and sprinkle with cumin seeds.
9. Preheat the oven to 365F. Put the tray with bagels in the oven and cook 30 minutes. Check if the bagels are cooked with the help of the toothpicks.
10. Cut the bagels and spread them with your favorite spread.

Nutrition: calories 262, fat 18.6, fiber 8.7, carbs 12, protein 15.1

Egg and Vegetable Hash

Preparation time: 8 minutes
Cooking time: 20 minutes
Servings: 6

Ingredients:

- 4 eggs
- 1 white onion, diced
- 6 oz turnip, chopped
- 2 bell peppers, chopped
- 1 garlic clove, peeled, diced
- 1 jalapeno pepper, sliced
- 5 oz Swiss cheese, grated
- 1 tablespoon lemon juice
- 1 tablespoon canola oil
- ½ teaspoon Taco seasoning

Directions:

1. Beat the eggs in the bowl and whisk gently.
2. Then pour canola oil in the pan and preheat it.
3. Add chopped turnips and white onion. Mix up the vegetables and cook them for 5 minutes over the medium heat. Stir them from time to time. Then add diced garlic and chopped peppers.
4. Sprinkle the vegetables with taco seasoning and mix up well.
5. Add lemon juice and close the lid. Cook it for 5 minutes more.
6. Then pour the whisked egg mixture over the vegetables. Sprinkle with the grated cheese.
7. Close the lid and cook it on the low heat for 10 minutes.
8. It is recommended to serve the dish hot.

Nutrition: calories 184, fat 12, fiber 1.5, carbs 8.7, protein 11

Cowboy Skillet

Preparation time: 5 minutes
Cooking time: 15 minutes
Servings: 4

Ingredients:

- 1 cup rutabaga, chopped
- 3 eggs, whisked
- ½ cup fresh cilantro, chopped
- 6 oz chorizo, chopped
- ½ teaspoon cayenne pepper
- 1 tablespoon olive oil
- ¾ cup heavy cream

Directions:

1. Put rutabaga in the skillet. Add olive oil and chorizo.
2. Mix the mixture up and close the lid. Cook it for 5 minutes over the medium heat.
3. When rutabaga becomes tender, add whisked eggs and chopped cilantro.
4. Add heavy cream and stir the meal with the help of a spatula.
5. Close the lid and sauté it for 10 minutes over the medium-low heat.

Nutrition: calories 362, fat 31.5, fiber 1, carbs 4.7, protein 15.4

Feta Quiche

Preparation time: 15 minutes
Cooking time: 25 minutes
Servings: 8
Ingredients:

- 8 oz Feta cheese, crumbled
- 5 eggs, whisked
- 1 cup spinach, chopped
- 1 garlic clove, diced
- 1 white onion, diced
- 1 teaspoon butter
- 5 oz Mozzarella, chopped
- ½ teaspoon chili flakes
- 1 teaspoon paprika
- ½ teaspoon white pepper
- ½ cup whipped cream

Directions:

1. Toss butter in the skillet and preheat it.
2. Add diced garlic and onion and cook it over the medium heat until the vegetables are soft.
3. Transfer the cooked vegetables in the mixing bowl. Add crumbled cheese, whisked eggs, spinach, chopped Mozzarella, chili flakes, paprika, white pepper, and whipped cream.
4. Mix the mixture well and transfer in the non-sticky mold. Flatten it gently with the spatula.
5. Place the mold in the preheated to 365f oven and cook quiche for 25 minutes.
6. Chill the quiche little and then cut into the servings.

Nutrition: calories 198, fat 14.7, fiber 0.5, carbs 4, protein 13

Bacon Pancakes

Preparation time: 10 minutes
Cooking time: 10 minutes
Servings: 2

Ingredients:

- 3 oz bacon, chopped
- ½ cup almond flour
- ¾ cup heavy cream
- ½ teaspoon baking powder
- ¼ teaspoon salt
- 1 egg, whisked

Directions:

1. Place the chopped bacon in the skillet and cook it for 5-6 minutes over the medium-high heat. The cooked bacon should be a little bit crunchy.
2. Meanwhile, mix up together almond flour, heavy cream, salt, baking powder, and whisked egg. When the mixture is smooth, the batter is cooked.
3. Add the cooked bacon in the batter and stir it gently with the help of the spoon.
4. Don't clean the skillet after t bacon. Ladle the bacon batter in the skillet and make the pancake.
5. Cook it for 1 minute from one side and then flip onto another side.
6. Cook it for 1.5 minutes more.
7. Make the same steps with the remaining batter.
8. Transfer the pancakes on the serving plate.

Nutrition: calories 458, fat 40.1, fiber 0.8, carbs 4.1, protein 20.9

Waffles

Preparation time: 10 minutes
Cooking time: 10 minutes
Servings: 4
Ingredients:
- 2 tablespoon butter, melted
- 4 eggs, whisked
- 1 teaspoon baking powder
- 1 teaspoon lemon juice
- 1 cup almond flour
- ½ teaspoon vanilla extract
- 1 tablespoon Erythritol
- ¾ cup organic almond milk

Directions:
1. In the mixing bowl combine together all the ingredients.
2. Whisk the smooth and homogenous batter.
3. Preheat the waffle maker well.
4. Pour enough of the batter in the waffle maker. Flatten it gently to get a waffle. Close it and cook until lightly golden.
5. Repeat the same steps with all remaining batter.
6. Serve the waffles warm.

Nutrition: calories 167, fat 13.7, fiber 1, carbs 3, protein 7.4

Chocolate Shake

Preparation time: 10 minutes

Cooking time: 5 minutes

Servings: 4

Ingredients:

- 2 cups heavy cream, whipped
- 1 tablespoon cocoa powder
- 1 tablespoon peanut butter
- ½ cup of coconut milk
- 2 tablespoons Erythritol
- ½ teaspoon vanilla extract

Directions:

1. Mix up together coconut milk and whipped heavy cream.
2. Add cocoa powder and mix it with the help of the hand mixer.
3. When the liquid is homogenous, add peanut butter, vanilla extract, and Erythritol.
4. Whisk it well.
5. Pour the chocolate shake in the serving glasses.

Nutrition: calories 304, fat 31.5, fiber 1.3, carbs 4.9, protein 3.2

Rolled Omelette with Mushrooms

Preparation time: 10 minutes
Cooking time: 20 minutes
Servings: 3
Ingredients:
- 1 cup mushrooms, chopped
- ½ white onion, sliced
- ½ teaspoon tomato paste
- 2 tablespoons water
- ½ teaspoon salt
- ½ teaspoon cayenne pepper
- ¾ teaspoon chili flakes
- 3 eggs, beaten
- 1 tablespoon cream cheese
- 1 teaspoon butter
- 1 teaspoon avocado oil

Directions:
1. Pour olive oil in the skillet and preheat it.
2. Add chopped mushrooms and sliced onion.
3. Then add tomato paste and water. Stir the ingredients and sauté them with the closed lid for 10 minutes.
4. Transfer the cooked vegetables in the mixing bowl.
5. Whisk together cream cheese, eggs, chili flakes, cayenne pepper, and salt.
6. Toss butter in the skillet and melt it.
7. Add egg mixture. Close the lid.
8. Cook it for 10 minutes over the medium-low heat.
9. Then spread the mushroom mixture over the cooked omelet and roll it.
10. Cut the cooked meal into 3 parts and transfer on the serving plates.

Nutrition: calories 102, fat 7.1, fiber 0.8, carbs 3.4, protein 6.8

Quiche Lorraine

Preparation time: 15 minutes
Cooking time: 18 minutes
Servings: 6

Ingredients:

- 1/3 cup butter, softened
- 1 cup almond flour
- ½ teaspoon salt
- 1 oz bacon, chopped
- 1 white onion, diced
- 1/3 cup heavy cream
- 5 oz Swiss cheese, grated
- 2 eggs, whisked
- ½ teaspoon ground black pepper
- 1 teaspoon olive oil

Directions:

1. Make the quiche crust: combine together softened butter, almond flour, and salt. Knead the dough. Roll it up.
2. Place it in the pie pan and flatten to get pie crust. Pin it with the help of the fork.
3. Preheat the oven to 360F and put the pan with pie crust inside. Cook it for 18 minutes.
4. Meanwhile, pour olive oil in the skillet.
5. Add diced onion and chopped bacon. Cook the ingredients for 5-6 minutes or until they are soft.
6. When the pie crust is cooked, remove it from the oven and chill little.
7. Spread it with the onion mixture and sprinkle with Swiss cheese.
8. Then combine together whisked eggs and heavy cream.
9. Pour the liquid over the cheese.
10. Transfer the pie in the oven and cook for 10 minutes at 355F.
11. Chill the cooked quiche well and cut into the servings.

Nutrition: calories 291, fat 25.8, fiber 0.9, carbs 4.5, protein 11.4

Breakfast Zucchini Bread

Preparation time: 15 minutes
Cooking time: 50 minutes
Servings: 8
Ingredients:

- ½ cup walnuts, chopped
- 1 teaspoon baking powder
- 1 tablespoon lemon juice
- 1 tablespoon flax meal
- 1 ½ cup almond flour
- 1 zucchini, grated
- 1 teaspoon xanthan gum
- 1 tablespoon butter, melted
- 3 eggs, beaten
- 1 teaspoon salt

Directions:

1. Preheat oven to 360F.
2. In the mixing bowl, combine all wet ingredients. Whisk the mixture well.
3. Then add baking powder, flax meal, almond flour, zucchini, xanthan gum, and salt. Mix up the mixture. Add chopped walnuts and stir it well. You will get a liquid but thick dough. Check if you add all the ingredients.
4. Transfer the dough into the non-sticky loaf mold and flatten its surface with the spatula.
5. Place the bread in the oven and cook for 50 minutes.
6. Check if the bread cooked with the help of the toothpick -if it is clean – the bread is cooked.
7. Remove the zucchini bread from the oven and chill well, then remove it from the mold and let it chill totally.
8. Slice it.

Nutrition: calories 123, fat 10.7, fiber 1.6, carbs 3.4, protein 5.6

Granola

Preparation time: 10 minutes
Cooking time: 25 minutes
Servings: 3

Ingredients:

- 4 tablespoons walnuts
- 3 tablespoons pecans
- 3 tablespoons hazelnuts
- 1 tablespoon chia seeds
- 2 tablespoons pumpkin seeds
- 2 tablespoons flax meal
- 1 tablespoon coconut shred
- 1 tablespoon Erythritol
- 2 tablespoons almond butter
- 1 tablespoon peanut butter

Directions:

1. Chop walnuts, pecans, hazelnuts, pumpkin seeds, and transfer in the mixing bowl.
2. Add chia seeds, flax meal coconut shred, Erythritol, almond butter, and peanut butter. Mix up the mixture. The mass should be sticky.
3. Preheat the oven to 300F.
4. Line the tray with parchment.
5. Transfer the nut mixture in the parchment and flatten it into the layer.
6. Place the tray in the oven and cook it for 25 minutes.
7. When the time is over, remove the tray from oven and chill granola.
8. Break it into medium size pieces. Store granola in the glass jar with the closed lid.

Nutrition: calories 373, fat 34.5, fiber 7.4, carbs 11.7, protein 11.6

Cheddar Souffle

Preparation time: 10 minutes
Cooking time: 25 minutes
Servings: 2
Ingredients:
- 2 oz Cheddar cheese, grated
- ½ teaspoon ground black pepper
- ½ teaspoon salt
- ½ cup almond milk
- ½ onion
- 1 bay leaf
- ¼ teaspoon peppercorn
- 1 tablespoon coconut shred
- 2 teaspoon butter, melted
- 2 eggs
- 1 teaspoon coconut oil
- ½ teaspoon paprika

Directions:
1. Brush the ramekins with coconut oil and sprinkle with coconut shred.
2. Then pour almond milk in the saucepan. Add onion and peppercorns.
3. Bring it to boil.
4. Remove onion and peppercorns.
5. Toss butter in the pan and add the almond flour. Stir it well until smooth.
6. Add salt, ground black pepper, and paprika. Mix up well.
7. After this, separate egg yolk and egg whites.
8. Add egg yolks in the almond flour mixture. Stir it well.
9. Add almond milk and start to preheat it. Stir it all the time until the mixture is smooth.
10. After this, whisk the egg whites till the strong peaks.
11. Add grated Cheddar in the almond flour mixture. Mix it up.
12. Then chill the mixture little.
13. Add egg whites and mix up gently.
14. Preheat the oven to 365F.
15. Place the cheese mixture into the prepared ramekins and transfer on the tray.

16. Put the tray in the preheated oven and cook for 15 minutes.
17. When the souffle is cooked, it will have a light brown color.

Nutrition: calories 384, fat 34.3, fiber 2.4, carbs 7.6, protein 14.5

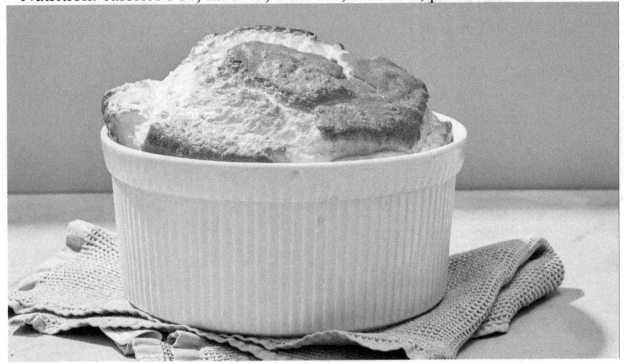

Mediterranean Omelette

Preparation time: 5 minutes
Cooking time: 10 minutes
Servings: 2
Ingredients:

- 3 eggs, beaten
- 1 tablespoon ricotta cheese
- 2 oz feta cheese, chopped
- 1 tomato, chopped
- 1 teaspoon butter
- ½ teaspoon salt
- 1 tablespoon scallions, chopped

Directions:

1. Mix up together ricotta cheese and eggs. Add salt and scallions.
2. Toss butter in the skillet and melt it.
3. Pour ½ part of whisked egg mixture in the skillet and cook it for 5-6 minutes or until it is solid -the omelet is cooked.
4. Then transfer omelet in the plate.
5. Make the second omelet with the remaining egg mixture.
6. Sprinkle each omelet with Feta and tomatoes. Roll them.

Nutrition: calories 203, fat 15.2, fiber 0.5, carbs 3.5, protein 13.6

Bacon Egg & Spinach Casserole

Preparation Time: 15 minutes
Cooking Time: 25 – 30 minutes
Servings: 2
Ingredients:

- 1/4 tsp. black pepper
- 1/3 green bell pepper, chopped
- 24 oz. spinach
- 3/4 cup cheddar, shredded
- 1 cup egg white
- 2/3 cup mushrooms, sliced
- 4 slices bacon, low sodium
- 2 tbsp. olive oil, separated
- 1/3 cup red onion, chopped
- olive oil cooking spray
- 1/4 tsp. salt
- 1 large egg
- 1/3 red bell pepper, chopped

Directions:

1. Scrub the bell pepper and mushrooms thoroughly. Chop the bell pepper and slice the mushrooms and set to the side.
2. Remove the outer skin from the onion and chop into small pieces. Set to the side.
3. Empty one tablespoon of the oil into a pan and arrange the sliced bacon, so they are not touching. Brown for approximately 2 minutes while flipping over as needed to fry to your preferred crispiness.
4. Transfer to a platter layered with kitchen paper and set to the side to cool.
5. Adjust your stove to heat at the temperature of 375° Fahrenheit. Apply olive oil to a glass baking dish and set to the side.
6. Transfer the 3 teaspoons of oil that remains into the skillet and combine the chopped mushrooms, onion, and bell pepper into the pan.
7. Heat for approximately three minutes. Half of the vegetables should be distributed using a slotted spoon on the prepped baking dish's base.

8. Layer the spinach over the vegetables and empty the remaining cooked vegetables on top of the spinach.
9. Use a glass dish to combine the pepper, egg, egg whites, and salt until integrated. Empty the dish on top of the cooked vegetables.
10. Take the cooked bacon, crush it into small chunks over the eggs, and dust it with the shredded cheese.
11. Heat in the stove for 20 minutes and remove to the counter.
12. Wait about a quarter of an hour before serving and enjoy!

Nutrition:
Calories: 248
Total Fat: 15g
Total Carbohydrates: 8g
Fiber: 3g
Sugar: 2g
Protein: 21g

Biscuits and Gravy

Preparation Time: 15 minutes
Cooking Time: 25 minutes
Servings: 2
Ingredients:

- 1 and 1/4 cups whole wheat flour, separated
- 1/2 tsp. Mrs. Dash's Table Blend, salt-free
- 2 tbsp. olive oil
- 1/4 tsp. black pepper
- 1 oz. margarine
- 1/2 tbsp. baking powder, salt-free
- 1/2 tsp. sugar, granulated
- 1/4 tsp. salt
- 1 and 1/2 cup milk, skim and separated

Directions:

1. Adjust the stove temperature to heat at 425° Fahrenheit. Layer a flat sheet with baking lining and set to the side.
2. Use a glass dish to blend the baking powder, one cup of the flour, seasoning, margarine, and granulated sugar until there is no more lumpiness present.
3. Finally, integrate 8 ounces of the milk into the mixture and blend until it becomes a thick dough.
4. Dust a flat surface with 2 tablespoons of the flour and flatten the pastry to be about one-inch thick.
5. Get a glass or a cookie cutter that is at least 2 inches in diameter, cut the dough into 6 individual circles.
6. Arrange on the prepped flat sheet and heat for approximately 14 minutes.
7. In the meantime, heat the olive oil, pepper, leftover 1/8 cup of flour, the leftover one-half cup of the skim milk, and salt in a skillet.
8. Warm gently for about 10 minutes as the gravy reduces while occasionally stirring.
9. Transfer the biscuits from the stove and move them onto individual serving plates.
10. Slice them in half and drizzle the gravy over the top.
11. Serve immediately and enjoy!

Nutrition:
Calories: 370 Total Fat: 21g
Total Carbohydrates: 34g Fiber: 1g
Sugar: 2g Protein: 14g

Breakfast Tostada

Preparation Time: 15 minutes
Cooking Time: 20 – 25 minutes
Servings: 2
Ingredients:

- 8 corn tortillas, low sodium
- 2 scallions, sliced thinly
- 8 tbsp. cream cheese, low-fat
- 1 tsp. Tabasco hot sauce
- 2 small tomatoes, deseeded and chopped
- 1 medium jalapeno, chopped
- 8 large eggs
- 2 slices Swiss cheese, low sodium
- 3 tbsp. cilantro, chopped
- olive oil cooking spray

Directions:

1. Set your stove to the temperature of 375° Fahrenheit.
2. Place the jalapeno pepper over the stove burner on the setting of a medium.
3. Flip the pepper over as it begins to turn black. This should take approximately 2 minutes.
4. Turn the burner off and move the jalapeno with the tongs to a paper towel for about 5 minutes.
5. In the meantime, arrange the tortillas onto the rack in the stove so they will not fall through.
6. Heat for approximately 6 minutes and remove carefully to serving dishes.
7. Put on a pair of gloves and rub the skin off of the jalapeno and chop finely. Set to the side.
8. Thoroughly wash the tomatoes and chop the scallions and tomatoes. Set aside.
9. Blend the cream cheese and Tabasco sauce in a glass dish until the consistency is smooth. Set to the side.
10. Coat a pan with the oil spray and heat the chopped jalapeno for about 90 seconds.

11. In a separate dish, whip the eggs and transfer the chopped scallions into the dish.
12. Empty the eggs into the skillet and occasionally stir the eggs to set for approximately 60 seconds.
13. Combine the chopped tomatoes and sliced cheese to the skillet and heat for another 2 minutes. Remove from the burner.
14. Evenly distribute the sour cream to each tortilla, spreading almost to the edges.

15.   Split the egg mixture evenly between each of the tortillas and serve immediately.

Nutrition:
Calories: 211
Total Fat: 8g
Total Carbohydrates: 22g
Fiber: 6g Sugar: 0.6g
Protein: 12g

Creamy Banana Oatmeal

Preparation Time: 5 minutes
Cooking Time: 10 minutes
Servings: 2
Ingredients:
- 1 cup of berries of choice
- 2 cups oats, old fashioned
- 1 and 1/3 cup almonds, sliced
- 3 and 1/4 cups water
- 1 tbsp. ground cinnamon
- 2 medium bananas

Directions:
1. Crush the bananas thoroughly until smooth.
2. Empty the water into a saucepan and incorporate the mashed banana.
3. Combine the oats in the pan and heat until the water bubbles.
4. Adjust the temperature of the burner to low and continue to warm for approximately 7 minutes.
5. Remove from heat and top with the ground cinnamon, berries, and sliced almonds.
6. Serve immediately and enjoy!

Nutrition:
Calories: 265
Total Fat: 3g
Total Carbohydrates: 47g
Fiber: 5g
Sugar: 0g
Protein: 15g

Egg Salad

Preparation Time: 10 minutes
Cooking Time: 15 minutes
Servings: 2
Ingredients:

- 1 and 1/2 cups pre-packaged salad greens
- 1/8-cup mozzarella cheese
- 1 cup sweet bell pepper of your choice, chopped
- 1/4 tsp. black pepper
- 1 tbsp. avocado, diced
- 2 large eggs
- 3/4 cup tomato, chopped
- 1/4 tsp. salt
- 8 cups cold water, separated
- 1 tsp. thyme, crushed
- 1/2 cup cucumber, sliced
- 1 tsp. olive oil

Directions:

1. Empty 4 cups of the cold water into a stockpot with the eggs and turn the burner on.
2. When the water starts to bubble, set a timer for 7 minutes.
3. Meanwhile, scrub and chop the tomato, cucumber, avocado, and bell pepper and transfer to a salad dish.
4. After the timer has chimed, remove the hot water and empty the remaining 4 cups of cold water on top of the eggs. Set aside for approximately 5 minutes.
5. Peel the shell once cooled and dice into small pieces then transfer to the dish.
6. Combine the salad greens and shredded mozzarella cheese to the salad dish and turn until integrated with the vegetables.
7. Dispense the olive oil over the dish and blend the crushed thyme, pepper, and salt until mixed well.
8. Serve immediately and enjoy!

Nutrition:
Calories: 200
Total Fat: 18g

Total Carbohydrates: 3g
Fiber: 0g
Sugar: 0g
Protein: 10g

Homemade Bacon

Preparation Time: 10 minutes
Cooking Time: 30 minutes
Servings: 2
Ingredients:
- 1 tsp. cumin seasoning
- 1 tsp. black pepper
- 2 tbsp. olive oil
- 16 oz. pork belly, sliced no more than 1/4 inch thick
- 4 tsp. liquid smoke
- 2 tsp. smoked paprika seasoning
- 3 tbsp. maple syrup
- 1/4 tsp. salt

Directions:
1. Set your stove to the temperature of 200° Fahrenheit. Cover a flat sheet with a rim with foil. Set to the side.
2. Remove the rind from the pork belly slices by using kitchen scissors and arrange the slices on the prepped baking pan, so they are in a single layer and not touching.
3. Utilize another pan if necessary, depending on the thickness of your bacon.
4. In a glass dish, blend the maple syrup and the liquid smoke until integrated.
5. In a separate dish, combine the pepper, cumin, and smoked paprika fully.
6. Use a pastry brush to apply the maple syrup to each of the bacon slices.
7. Turn the slices over and repeat step 5.
8. Dust all of the slices with the mixed seasonings and rub the spices into the meat.
9. Empty the olive oil into a skillet and arrange the slices in a single layer. You will need to cook in stages.
10. Brown for approximately 2 minutes while turning over as needed to fry to your desired crispiness fully.
11. Arrange to the plate and enjoy while hot!

Nutrition:
Calories: 145
Total Fat: 15g
Total Carbohydrates: 0g
Fiber: 0g
Sugar: 0g
Protein: 3g

Oatmeal Pancakes

Preparation Time: 10 minutes
Cooking Time: 20 minutes
Servings: 2
Ingredients:

- 1/2 tsp. ground cinnamon
- 4 oz. whole wheat flour
- 2 oz. oats, old fashioned
- 1 tsp. baking powder, salt-free
- 1/8 tsp. salt
- olive oil cooking spray
- 4 oz. milk, skim
- 1/8-cup Greek yogurt, no-fat
- 1 large egg
- 1/2 tsp. vanilla extract
- 3 tsp. brown sugar

Directions:

1. In a big dish, blend the salt, whole wheat flour, ground cinnamon, and whole oats, and baking powder, combine completely.
2. Using another dish, fully integrate the milk and egg until the mixed well.
3. Combine the vanilla extract, yogurt, and brown sugar into the eggs and whisk to remove any lumpiness.
4. Slowly empty the egg dish into the flour dish, making sure it is combined but do not mix too thoroughly.
5. Warm a skillet. Make sure the skillet is sprayed with olive oil.
6. Distribute approximately a quarter of the batter into the skillet.
7. Turn the pancake over after the top starts to bubble after about 60 seconds.
8. Let the pancake cook for approximately another minute and flip as needed until browned completely.
9. Remove to a plate and coat the skillet with an additional coat of olive oil spray.
10. Repeat until all the pancakes are finished.
11. Serve while hot and enjoy!

Nutrition:

Calories: 196
Total Fat: 2g
Total Carbohydrates: 32g
Fiber: 4g
Sugar: 2g
Protein: 10g

Sausage and Potatoes Mix

Preparation time: 10 minutes

Cooking time: 22 minutes

Servings: 2

Ingredients:

- 1/2-pound smoked sausage, cooked and chopped
- 3 tablespoons olive oil
- 3/4-pounds red potatoes, cubed
- yellow onions, chopped
- 1 teaspoon thyme, dried
- 2 teaspoons cumin, ground
- A pinch of black pepper

Directions:

1. Warm-up a pan using the oil over medium-high heat, add potatoes and onions, stir and cook for 12 minutes.
2. Supply sausage, thyme, cumin, and black pepper, stir, cook for 10 minutes more, divide between plates and serve for lunch.
3. Enjoy!

Nutrition:

Calories: 199 Total Fat: 2g

Total Carbohydrates: 14g

Fiber: 4g Sugar: 0g Protein: 8g

Nice Wheat Muffins

Preparation Time: 10 minutes
Cooking Time: 25 minutes
Servings: 2
Ingredients:

- cooking spray
- 2 cups whole wheat flour
- 1/2 cup of sugar
- 3 1/2 tsps. baking powder
- 2 egg whites
- 3 Tbsps. canola oil
- 1/3 cups fat-free milk
- Tbsp. white vinegar (add this towards the nonfat milk and stir well)
- Optional: 1 cup blueberries, fresh or frozen

Directions:

1. Preheat the oven to 350°F.
2. Insert paper lines right into a muffin tray.
3. Place the flour, baking powder, sugar within a bowl, and mix well.
4. If the blueberries should be added, fold the fruits into the batter since it will avoid the fruits engaging in the bowl's bottom. Leave aside.
5. In another bowl, mix in the total amount of ingredients.
6. Fold the flour mixture, combine well without over-mixing.
7. Fold the batter into the muffin cups and place it within the oven.
8. Bake for approximately 25 minutes before muffins are well cooked.

Nutrition:
Calories: 134
Total Fat: 1.4g
Total Carbohydrates: 27g
Fiber: 4g
Sugar: 5g
Protein: 6g

Pumpkin Vanilla Smoothie

Preparation Time: 5 minutes
Cooking Time: 5 minutes
Servings: 2
Ingredients:

- cup milk
- Tbsps. unsweetened instant tea (optional)
- 1/2 tsp. pumpkin pie spice
- 1/4 tsp. ground cardamom
- 1 banana
- 3/4 cup fat -free vanilla yogurt
- 1/2 cup canned pumpkin
- 1 Tbsp. pure maple syrup
- 1 cup ice (about 10 cubes)

Directions:

1. Place the moment tea as well as the spices inside a food processor.
2. Mix inside the milk and process before tea is well dissolved.
3. Toss in the total amount ingredients, excluding the ice and blend until smooth.
4. Depending on the thickness, continue adding ice to find you in the right consistency.
5. Transfer the mixture into individual glasses and serve.

Nutrition:
Calories: 175 Total Fat: 0g
Total Carbohydrates: 15g
Fiber: 5g Sugar: 7g
Protein: 23g

Pumpkin Pie Smoothie Delight

Preparation Time: 5 minutes

Cooking Time: 5 minutes

Servings: 2

Ingredients:

- 1 scoop vanilla whey protein
- 1/4 cup 100% pumpkin purees (NOT pie filling!)
- 1/8 cup Splenda granular
- 1 Dash salt (I take advantage of Morton' s Lite Salt)
- pumpkin pie spice, to taste
- 1 cup of soy milk
- 2 Tbsps. Fat-Free Cool Whip
- 4-5 ice, if desired

Directions:

1. Place all ingredients inside a food processor.
2. Add all the ingredients, and then mix until smooth.
3. Add the ice, if required.

Nutrition:

Calories: 150

Total Fat: 2g

Total Carbohydrates: 28g

Fiber: 6g

Sugar: 6g

Protein: 15g

Buckwheat Pancakes with Strawberries

Preparation Time: 5 minutes
Cooking Time: 15 minutes
Servings: 2
Ingredients

- 2 Egg whites
- 1 tablespoon Olive oil
- 1/2 cup Fat-free milk
- 1/2 cup All-purpose flour
- 1/2 cup Buckwheat flour
- 1 tablespoon Baking powder
- 1/2 cup Sparkling normal water
- 2 cups sliced Fresh strawberries

Directions:

1. Mix the egg whites, olive oil, and milk in a big bowl.
2. In another bowl combine the all-purpose flour, buckwheat flour, and baking powder and mix thoroughly.
3. Slowly add the dry ingredients towards the egg white mixture while you alternately add the dazzling water. Be sure to mix between each addition until all the ingredients combine right into a batter.
4. Warm a non-stick frying pan on medium heat. Spoon 1/2 cup of the pancake batter into the pan. Cook before top surface in the pancake bubbles plus the edges turns lightly brown, about 2 minutes.
5. Flip and cook before the bottom are nicely brown and cooked through, one to two minutes longer. Repeat with the other pancake batter. Transfer the pancakes to individual plates. Top each with 1/2 cup sliced strawberries. Serve.

Nutrition:
Calories: 142 Total Fat: 3g
Total Carbohydrates: 25g Fiber: 4g Sugar: 6g
Protein: 6g

Triple Muffins

Preparation Time: 10 minutes
Cooking Time: 25 minutes
Servings: 2
Ingredients:

- non-stick cooking spray
- 1-1/3 cups all-purpose flour
- 3/4 cup buckwheat flour
- 1/4 to 1/3 cup sugar
- 1-1/2 tsp. baking powder
- 1 tsp. ground cinnamon
- 1/2 tsp. baking soda
- 1/2 tsp. salt
- 2 eggs, slightly beaten
- 1 cup mashed cooked butternut squash
- 1/2 cup fat-free milk
- 2 Tbsps. cooking oil
- 1/2 tsp. finely shredded orange peel
- 1/4 cup orange juice
- 3/4 cup fresh or frozen blueberries
- 1 Rolled oats

Directions:

1. Preheat the oven to 400°F.
2. Insert paper liners right into a 12 x 2 1/2- inches muffin cups and leave aside.
3. Add the flours, baking powder, baking soda, sugar, and salt in a mixing bowl. Mix well.
4. Dig a proper in the center of the mixture and keep aside for some time.
5. Mix the eggs milk, squash, oil, orange juice, plus the peel in another bowl.
6. Put the flour mixture into the egg mixture and mix until moist.
7. Mix inside the blueberries.
8. Fold the batter mixture into the lined muffin cups and top up each cup with oats.
9. Bake for approximately 20 minutes before muffins certainly are a light brown.

10.   Allow cooling for 5-6 minutes.
11.   Take right out of the muffin cups and serve.
Nutrition:
Calories: Total Fat: g
Total Carbohydrates: g Fiber: g
Sugar: g Protein: g

Pineapple Potato Salad

Preparation time: 10 minutes
Cooking time: 30 minutes
Servings: 2
Ingredients:
- 2 cups pineapple, peeled and cubed
- 4 sweet potatoes, cubed
- 1 tablespoon olive oil
- 1/4 cup coconut, unsweetened and shredded
- 1/3 cup almonds, chopped
- 1 cup coconut cream

Directions:
1. Arrange sweet potatoes on the lined baking sheet, add the olive oil.
2. Introduce within the oven at 350°F.
3. Roast for 30 minutes; put them in a salad bowl.
4. Add coconut, pineapple, almonds, and cream, toss.
5. Split between plates and serve as a side dish. Enjoy!

Nutrition:
Calories: 150
Total Fat: 0.3g
Total Carbohydrates: 36g
Fiber: 3g
Sugar: 14g
Protein: 2g

Breakfast Sausage Gravy

Preparation Time: 5 minutes
Cooking Time: 15 minutes
Servings: 2
Ingredients:

- 1/2 lb. ground breakfast sausage
- 1/4 cup all-purpose flour
- 3 cups of milk
- Salt
- Pepper to taste

Directions:

1. Place the bottom breakfast sausages on the non-stick skillet.
2. Leave for approximately 7-8 minutes until they may be well browned.
3. Contribute the flour, milk, salt, pepper, and stir well.
4. Let the mixture boil and thicken for some time.
5. Lower heat and leave for 4-5 minutes.
6. Serve.

Nutrition:
Calories: 138
Total Fat: 8g
Total Carbohydrates: 7g
Fiber: 0g
Sugar: 3g
Protein: 8g

Bisquick Turkey Breakfast Balls

Preparation Time: 5 minutes
Cooking Time: 25 – 30 minutes
Servings: 2
Ingredients:

- 16 oz. cheddar 2%
- 3 cups heart healthy Bisquick
- 16 oz. low sodium turkey breakfast sausage
- 1/3 cup milk

Directions:

1. Preheat an oven to 375°F.
2. Place all ingredients within a bowl.
3. Add more Bisquick if the mixture is too sticky.
4. Form little round balls and put on a cookie sheet.
5. Bake for approximately quarter-hour until cooked.
6. Allow to cool and serve.

Nutrition:
Calories: 224
Total Fat: 5g
Total Carbohydrates: 16g
Fiber: 11g
Sugar: 2g
Protein: 14g

Easy Omelet Waffles

Preparation time: 10 minutes
Cooking time: 5 minutes
Servings: 2
Ingredients:
- 4 eggs
- A pinch of black pepper
- 2 tablespoons ham, chopped
- 1/4 cup low-fat cheddar, shredded
- 2 tablespoons parsley, chopped
- Cooking spray

Directions:
1. Within a bowl, combine the eggs with pepper, ham, cheese, and parsley and whisk effectively.
2. Grease your waffle iron with cooking spray, add the eggs mix, cook for 4-5 minutes.
3. Divide the waffles between plates and serve them for breakfast.
4. Enjoy!

Nutrition:
Calories: 200
Total Fat: 7g
Total Carbohydrates: 29g
Fiber: 3g
Sugar: 0g
Protein: 3g

Breakfast Fruit Bowl
Preparation time: 5 minutes
Cooking time: 5 minutes
Servings: 2
Ingredients:
- cup mango, chopped
- 1 banana, sliced
- 1 cup pineapple, chopped
- 1 cup almond milk

Directions:
1. Prepare a bowl, combine the mango using the banana, pineapple, and almond milk.
2. Stir, divide into smaller bowls, and serve breakfast.
3. Enjoy!

Nutrition:
Calories: 103
Total Fat: 0g
Total Carbohydrates: 25g
Fiber: 0g
Sugar: 0g
Protein: 1g

CHAPTER 5:

Lunch

Curried Chicken wrap

Preparation Time: 10 minutes
Cooking Time: 10 minutes
Servings: 2
Ingredients:
- 2 medium whole-wheat tortilla
- 1/3 cup cooked chicken, chopped
- 1 cup apple, chopped
- 1 tablespoon light mayonnaise
- 1 teaspoon curry powder
- 1 cup, or about 15, raw baby carrots

Directions:
1. Mix together all the ingredients except tortillas.
2. Divide and place at the center of the tortillas.
3. Roll and serve.

Nutrition:
Calories: 380
Total Fat: 9g
Total Carbohydrates: 47g
Fiber: 4g
Sugar: 5g
Protein: 27g

Open-Faced Garden Tuna Sandwich

Preparation Time: 10 minutes
Cooking Time: 15 minutes
Servings: 2
Ingredients:

- 2 cans (5 ounces each) low sodium tuna packed in water, drained
- 4 green onions, sliced
- 4 slices hearty multigrain bread
- 1 tablespoon fresh parsley, chopped
- 1 tablespoon lemon juice
- 1 tablespoon extra-virgin olive oil
- 1/4 cup cherry tomatoes, sliced
- A handful of fresh arugulas
- 2 tablespoons low fat whipped cream cheese - Black pepper powder to taste

Directions:

1. Mix together oil, lemon juice, parsley, green onion, and pepper.
2. Add tuna to a bowl. Add about 2/3 of the above mixture and mix well.
3. Spread a little of the remaining mixture lightly on both sides of the bread.
4. Heat a nonstick pan over high heat. Place the bread slices and cook until the bottom side is golden brown. Turn and cook the other side. Add the remaining mixture to the arugula and toss well. To make sandwiches: Spread cream cheese on each of the bread slices. Divide and spread the tuna mixture over the slices. Place the arugula over the tuna mixture and finally cherry tomatoes.

Nutrition:
Calories: 360 Total Fat: 20g
Total Carbohydrates: 18g Fiber: 5g
Sugar: 5g Protein: 24g

Baked Macaroni

Preparation Time: 10 minutes
Cooking Time: 30 minutes
Servings: 2
Ingredients:
- 1-pound extra-lean ground beef
- 2 large onions, diced
- 2 boxes (7 ounces each) whole-wheat elbow macaroni, cooked according to instructions on the package
- 2 jars (15 ounces each) low sodium spaghetti sauce
- 3/4 cup Parmesan cheese

Directions:
1. Prepare a large nonstick pan over medium heat. Add onions and sauté for a few minutes until the onions are translucent.
2. Add beef and cook until brown. Add pasta and spaghetti sauce. Mix well and transfer into a greased baking dish.
3. Bake in a preheated oven at 350 degrees F for about 30 minutes.
4. Serve garnished with Parmesan cheese.

Nutrition:
Calories: 200
Total Fat: 7g
Total Carbohydrates: 25g
Fiber: 0g
Sugar: 3g
Protein: 4g

Zucchini Pad Thai

Preparation Time: 15 minutes
Cooking Time: 30 minutes
Servings: 2
Ingredients:
For the sauce:

- 3/4 tablespoon coconut sugar
- 1 teaspoon Sriracha sauce or to taste
- 2 tablespoons tamarind paste
- 2 teaspoons low sodium tamari
- 1 tablespoon lime juice
- 2 tablespoons low sodium chicken stock

For the noodles:

- large carrot, peeled, trimmed with top and bottom sliced off
- 2 large zucchinis, trimmed with top and bottom sliced off

For Pad Thai:

- 1/2 cups bean sprouts
- 1 large skinless, boneless chicken breast, sliced
- 1 egg, beaten
- 2 teaspoons olive oil, divided
- 1 green onion, thinly sliced
- 2 tablespoons peanuts, finely chopped
- Lime wedges to serve
- Salt to taste
- Pepper powder to taste

Directions:

1. To make noodles: Make noodles of the carrot and zucchini using a spiralizer or a julienne peeler.
2. For pad Thai: Place a nonstick pan over medium heat. Add 1/2-teaspoon oil. When the oil is heated, add egg, salt, and pepper. Keep stirring to scramble it. Remove from the pan when cooked and place it in a bowl.
3. Put oil in a warm nonstick pan. Once heated, add chicken breasts, salt, and pepper.
4. Cook until the chicken is tender inside and golden-brown outside. Place it along with the egg.

5. To make the sauce: Add all the ingredients of the sauce to a bowl and mix well. Place the pan back on the heat. Put the sauce mixture into the pan and cook until it is bubbly.
6. Add zucchini and carrot noodles and cook sauté for a few minutes until it is thoroughly heated and slightly softened.
7. Add chicken, eggs, and sprouts. Mix well and heat thoroughly.

8. Garnish with lemon wedges, green onion, and peanuts and serve immediately.

Nutrition:
Calories: 224
Total Fat: 3g
Total Carbohydrates: 12g
Fiber: 6g
Sugar: 10g
Protein: 11g

Easy Roasted Salmon

Preparation Time: 5 minutes

Cooking Time: 25 minutes

Servings: 2

Ingredients:

- 8 (6 ounces each) wild salmon fillets
- 2 lemons, cut into 8 wedges
- Freshly ground black pepper to taste
- 1/2 cup fresh dill, minced
- 8 cloves garlic, peeled and minced

Directions:

1. Lay the salmon fillets in a large greased baking dish. Sprinkle lemon juice, pepper, dill, and garlic.
2. Prepare the oven at 400 degrees F then place the dish and bake for about 20-25 minutes until the salmon is opaque.
3. Serve immediately.

Nutrition:

Calories: 240 Total Fat: 14g

Total Carbohydrates: 0g

Fiber: 0g Sugar: 0g Protein: 28g

Shrimp with Pasta, Artichoke, and Spinach

Preparation Time: 10 minutes
Cooking Time: 30 minutes
Servings: 2
Ingredients:
- 1 tablespoon grapeseed oil
- 1 medium onion, diced small
- 1/2 cup mushrooms, thinly sliced
- 2 garlic cloves, thinly sliced
- 1/2 cup canned artichokes, quartered
- 1/2 cups chicken broth
- 6-ounce raw angel hair pasta, broken in half
- 1/2 cup raw shrimps, peeled, deveined
- 1/2 teaspoon dried oregano
- 1/2 cup fresh spinach roughly chopped
- Salt to taste
- Pepper to taste

Optional:
- A pinch of crushed red pepper flakes

Directions:
1. Place a pot with oil over medium heat. When the oil is heated, add onions, mushrooms, and garlic.
2. Sauté for a couple of minutes and add artichokes, chicken broth, pasta, shrimps, oregano, red pepper flakes, salt, and pepper.
3. Mix well and bring to a boil. Put cover and cook until the pasta is al dente.
4. Add spinach and cook for a couple of minutes until the spinach wilts.
5. Adjust the seasonings if required. Serve hot.

Nutrition:
Calories: 500
Total Fat: 18g
Total Carbohydrates: 56g
Fiber: 12g
Sugar: 0g
Protein: 30g

Pistachio Crusted Halibut with Spicy Yogurt

Preparation Time: 15 minutes
Cooking Time: 30 minutes
Servings: 2
Ingredients:
For Halibut

- 6 (1 1/4-inch-thick) pieces skinless halibut fillet of about 6 ounces each
- 1/2 cup shelled pistachio nuts (chopped)
- 1/2 cups whole milk
- 1/3 cup extra virgin olive oil
- 4 1/2 tablespoons cornmeal
- 1/2 tsp. black pepper powder (to taste)

For spicy yogurt:

- 1/2 cups thick Greek yogurt
- 1 cup cucumber, peeled, finely chopped
- 1 medium onion, finely chopped
- 2 tablespoons fresh dill, chopped
- 2 tablespoons lemon juice
- 2 teaspoons dried Maras pepper
- 3/4 teaspoon salt

Directions:

1. Place fish in a baking dish. Pour milk all over the fish. Put cover and refrigerate about 30 minutes.
2. Meanwhile, mix in shallow bowl pistachio nuts and cornmeal.
3. Get the fish with a slotted spoon and place on a plate. Season with salt and pepper. Coat the fish pieces with cornmeal mixture and place them on another plate.
4. Place a heavy skillet over medium-high heat. Add oil. When the oil is heated, place the fish pieces in it. When the underside is golden, flip sides and cook the other side of the fish until golden brown.
5. Meanwhile make the spicy yogurt as follows: Mix all the Ingredients of spicy yogurt and set aside.
6. Serve fried fish with spicy yogurt.

Nutrition:
Calories: 232

Total Fat: 8g
Total Carbohydrates: 5g
Fiber: 0g
Sugar: 0g
Protein: 31g

Paella with Chicken, Leeks, and Tarragon

Preparation Time: 15 minutes

Cooking Time: 20 minutes

Servings: 2

Ingredients:

- 2 teaspoons extra-virgin olive oil
- 1 large onion, sliced
- 4 leeks (whites only), thinly sliced
- 6 -7 garlic cloves, minced
- 1 pound's chicken breast, boneless, skinless, cut into strips of 1/2-inch-wide and 2 inches' long
- 1 large tomato, chopped
- 1 red pepper, sliced
- 1 green pepper, sliced
- 1 1/3 cups long-grain brown rice
- 2 teaspoons tarragon, or to taste
- 2 cups fat-free, unsalted chicken broth
- 2 cups frozen peas
- 1/2 cup chopped fresh parsley
- 2 lemons, cut into 4 wedges each

Directions:

1. Put olive oil in a skillet with medium temperature. Once heated, sauté onions, garlic, leeks, and chicken for a few minutes or until the onions are translucent and the chicken is light brown.
2. Add tomatoes, peppers, and sauté for 4-5 minutes.
3. Add rice, tarragon, and broth. Mix well.
4. When it boils, lower heat, cover, and simmer for about 12-15 minutes.
5. Uncover and add peas. Wait for it to simmer or until all the moisture is absorbed and rice is cooked.
6. Sprinkle parsley and serve with lemon wedges.

Nutrition:

Calories: 378

Total Fat: 6g

Total Carbohydrates: 46g

Fiber: 7g

Sugar: 0g

Protein: 35g

Roasted Brussels Sprouts, Chicken, and Potatoes

Preparation Time: 10 minutes

Cooking Time: 20 minutes

Servings: 2

Ingredients:

- 1/2-pound chicken breasts, boneless, skinless, cut into 2 pieces
- 1/2 cups Yukon gold potatoes or red potatoes, cut into bite-sized pieces
- 2 cups Brussels sprouts, trimmed, quartered
- 1/2 cup onions, diced
- 1/4 cup vinaigrette dressing
- 1 tablespoon lemon juice
- 1/4 teaspoon garlic salt
- 1 teaspoon dried oregano
- 1 teaspoon Dijon mustard
- 2 tablespoons Kalamata olives, quartered
- Freshly ground black pepper to taste
- Cooking spray

Directions:

1. Grease a baking sheet with cooking spray.
2. Place the chicken pieces, Brussels sprouts, potatoes, and onions in a large bowl.
3. Mix together in a small bowl: vinaigrette, lemon juice, mustard, oregano, pepper, olives, and garlic salt and put vegetables in the bowl.
4. Transfer the contents to the baking sheet.
5. Bake in a warm oven at 400 degrees F for 20 minutes or until the chicken and potatoes are tender.
6. Stir in between a couple of times.
7. Remove from the oven. Mix well and serve.

Nutrition:

Calories: 361 Total Fat: 10g

Total Carbohydrates: 37g

Fiber: 7g Sugar: 0g Protein: 32g

Shepherd's Pie

Preparation Time: 10 minutes
Cooking Time: 30 minutes
Servings: 2
Ingredients:

- 1 large baking potato, peeled, diced
- 1/4 cup low-fat milk
- 1/2-pound lean ground beef
- 1 medium onion, chopped
- 2 cloves garlic, minced
- 1 tablespoon flour
- 2 cups of frozen mixed vegetables
- 1/2 cup low sodium beef broth
- 1/2 cup cheddar cheese, sliced
- Pepper powder to taste

Directions:

1. Prepare a saucepan covered with water then put the potatoes. Cook until the potatoes are done. Drain and mash the potatoes.
2. Add milk to the mashed potatoes and mix well. Keep aside
3. Place a skillet over medium heat. Add onion, garlic, and beef. Cook until the beef is browned.
4. Add vegetables and broth. Heat thoroughly.
5. Transfer to a baking dish. Spread the potato mixture over this.
6. Sprinkle cheese on top.
7. Bake in a warm oven at 375 degrees for 25 -30 minutes or until the cheese is lightly browned.

Nutrition:
Calories: 420
Total Fat: 21g
Total Carbohydrates: 29g
Fiber: 3g
Sugar: 5g
Protein: 28g

Salmon and Edamame Cakes

Preparation Time: 10 minutes
Cooking Time: 30 minutes
Servings: 2
Ingredients:

- 4 cups flaked, cooked salmon
- 1 cup frozen edamame, thawed
- 4 large egg whites
- 1/2 cup whole-wheat panko breadcrumbs (Japanese breadcrumbs)
- 2 scallions, finely chopped
- 2 tablespoons fresh ginger, peeled, minced
- 2 cloves garlic, crushed
- 2 tablespoons cilantro, finely chopped
- Canola oil cooking spray
- Lime wedges to serve

Directions:

1. Add all the Ingredients except lime wedges to a bowl and mix well.
2. Divide the mixture into 8-10 balls and shape them into cakes.
3. Arrange the cakes on a wax paper-lined plate. Refrigerate the cakes for about 30 minutes.
4. Place a nonstick skillet over medium heat. Spray with cooking spray. When the skillet is heated, place the cakes 3-4 cakes.
5. Cook until the underside is golden brown. Flip and cook the other side.
6. Serve hot with lemon wedges and a dip of your choice.

Nutrition:
Calories: 267
Total Fat: 13g
Total Carbohydrates: 5g
Fiber: 1g
Sugar: 0g
Protein: 21g

Flat Bread Pizza

Preparation Time: 5 minutes
Cooking Time: 20 minutes
Servings: 2
Ingredients:

- 1 tbsp. of olive oil, plus topping if needed
- 1 lb. flatbread dough (use the whole-grain dough while on a DASH diet)
- 1/2 tsp of dried herbs, red pepper flakes, or other needed spices
- 1 bunch of fresh broccoli, cauliflower, arugula, or other leafy greens vegetables
- 1 bell pepper, diced

Directions:

1. Set the grill to medium heat and brush a thin oil layer.
2. Cook the flatbread dough on both sides until golden brown, about 2 minutes on either side.
3. Top flatbread with freshly sliced vegetables and green vegetables. Season to taste, using olive oil, salt, pepper, red pepper flakes, or herbs.
4. To finish cooking, relocate flatbread pizza to the oven.

Nutrition:
Calories: 130
Total Fat: 1g
Total Carbohydrates: 25g
Fiber: 0g
Sugar: 2g
Protein: 5g

Spinach Salad with Walnuts and Strawberry

Preparation Time: 10 minutes
Cooking Time: 15 minutes
Servings: 2
Ingredients:
- 1/2 cup walnuts
- 4 cups of fresh spinach, loosely trimmed stems
- 3 tbsp. of honey
- 2 tbsp. of spicy brown mustard
- 1/4 cup of balsamic vinegar
- 1/4 tsp of sea salt
- 1/4 cup of crumbled feta (about 1 oz.), optional

Directions:
1. Heat the oven until 375 ° F.
2. Arrange walnuts on a rimmed baking sheet and bake for 8 minutes, until they are fragrant and toasted. Switch to a cool plate.
3. Place the spinach in a large container. The honey, mustard, vinegar, and salt are whisked together in a small cup.
4. Drizzle the salad over 3/4 of the dressing and scatter the walnuts on top.
5. Serve sprinkled with both the cheese (if it is used) and the remaining side dressing.

Nutrition:
Calories: 129
Total Fat: 8g
Total Carbohydrates: 10g
Fiber: 3g
Sugar: 0.8g
Protein: 6.6g

Chicken Vegetable Soup

Preparation Time: 5 minutes
Cooking Time: 10 – 15 minutes
Servings: 2
Ingredients:

- 2 tbsp. of olive oil
- 3 garlic cloves
- 1 onion
- 4 cups of low sodium chicken broth
- 1/2 cup of carrot, sliced
- 1/2 cup of a parsnip, sliced
- 2 cups of a green collar, minced
- 1 can of black beans, drained
- 1/2 cup of seaweed (optional)

Directions:

1. Simmer in the olive oil, garlic, and onion blended.
2. Pour the broth and vegetables into the chicken and turn to a boil. Switch to a simmer when boiling.
3. Keep on simmer until the vegetables are soft.
4. Pour in the strained canned beans and optional seaweed when 5 minutes left to cook.

Nutrition:
Calories: 120
Total Fat: 4g
Total Carbohydrates: 11g
Fiber: 2g
Sugar: 4g
Protein: 10g

Avocado Sandwich with Lemon and Cilantro

Preparation Time: 10 minutes
Cooking Time: 10 minutes
Servings: 2
Ingredients:
- 1 medium Hass avocado
- 2 slices of 100% whole wheat bread
- 1/2 cup spinach
- 1/4 cup cilantro
- 1/2 carrots
- 1/4 cup cucumber
- 1/4 cup blueberries
- 1/4 cup red cherries
- 1 tbsp. lemon juice
- 1 cup skim milk

Directions:
1. Toast the bread.
2. Slice the avocado (or as desired) into thin strips and put on toast.
3. Slice the vegetables, then put them on toast.
4. Sprinkle with a splash of salt and lemon juice.
5. Prepare the fruit and enjoy a bowl of mixed fruit on the side with skim milk.

Nutrition:
Calories: 580 Total Fat: 31g
Total Carbohydrates: 50g
Fiber: 4g Sugar: 0g Protein: 9g

Tofu and Mushroom Burger

Preparation Time: 10 minutes
Cooking Time: 15 minutes
Servings: 2
Ingredients:

- 6 oz. solid tofu
- 4 oz. mushrooms
- 1 medium onion, chopped
- 1 medium red onion, chopped
- 2 cloves of garlic, minced
- 1 medium tomatoes, diced
- 1 oz. cheese (your preference)
- 1 oz. coriander, cut
- 1 chili, finely grated
- 1 egg, beaten
- 1 tbsp. of flour
- 1 tbsp. of canola oil
- 2 whole-wheat hamburger buns
- salt and pepper, to taste
- 1 lettuce - ketchup
- 1 tbsp. of flour
- 4 tbsp. of canola oil

Directions:

1. Preheat oven to 275 degrees F.
2. Sauté the onions, garlic, chili, and mushrooms in a saucepan under medium-high heat. Put it aside.
3. Then add the tofu, mushrooms, cilantro, and mash together with a fork in a pot.
4. Add the flour and the egg and blend well in a malleable consistency. Shape into the patties. Fry patties on both sides in a pan under medium heat, until golden brown. Put it in the oven for 5 minutes.
5. Place the cheese on the burgers, turn off the oven, and allow the cheese to melt over the burger. Serve, and have fun!

Nutrition:
Calories: 400 Total Fat: 12g
Total Carbohydrates: 60g Fiber: 5g

Sugar: 0g Protein: 16g

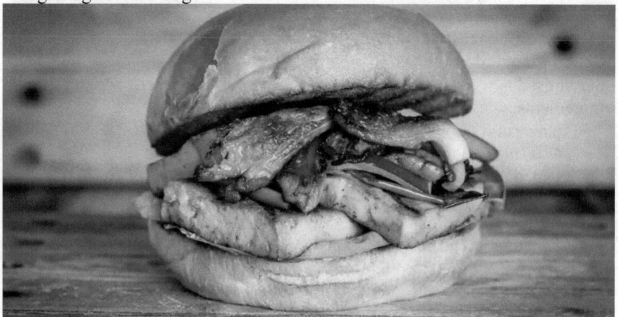

Cobb Salad

Preparation Time: 10 minutes
Cooking Time: 15 – 20 minutes
Servings: 2
Ingredients:
- 2 tbsp. extra virgin olive oil
- 2 skinless, boneless breast chicken halves (about 1 lb.), pounded thin with a meat tenderizer instrument
- 1/4 cup leftover roasted turkey breast
- 1 lb. head roman lettuce, sliced, rinsed and spin-dried
- small bunch of frisée or your choice of lettuce if not available, divided, washed, and spun dry
- 1 medium avocado, pitted, peeled, and chopped
- 3 large eggs, hard-boiled and chopped into circles
- 1 tbsp. chopped mustard seed
- 1 tbsp. sliced fresh chives
- 1 tbsp. freshly squeezed lemon juice
- freshly chopped black pepper (optional)

Directions:
1. Warm the cooking oil over medium heat in a cast-iron skillet.
2. Pat the chicken breasts with paper towels and cook for 6 to 8 minutes, flipping halfway through. Test an internal temperature of 160 ° F with an instant-read thermometer. Remove from heat, arrange on a plate, cover with foil loosely, and put aside.
3. Attach the diced turkey to the same pan and cook for 2 to 3 minutes, just enough to crisp. Remove the paper towels from the heat and rinse.
4. Combine the romaine then frisée, then put on two wide plates equally. Slice the chicken, then place it on top.
5. Arrange the turkey, avocado, tomato, and chopped eggs over the lettuce in orderly rows.
6. The lemon juice, mustard seed, and chives are mixed in a small cup. Put the glaze on top of the salad, if needed, supplemented with pepper.

Nutrition:
Calories: 400 Total Fat: 28g
Total Carbohydrates: 12g

Fiber: g5 Sugar: 4g
Protein: 30g

Veggie Sushi

Preparation Time: 10 minutes
Cooking Time: 15 minutes
Servings: 2
Ingredients:

- 3 cups of brown rice
- 2 tbsp. of rice wine vinegar
- 2 avocados, longitudinally cut
- 2 carrots, longitudinally sliced
- 1 cucumber, longitudinally sliced
- Ponzu sauce, to taste

Directions:

1. Cook brown rice, as indicated in instructions. Fold rice to vinegar rice wine. Let the cooked rice cool down.
2. When cool, spread rice uniformly with a wooden spoon on a bamboo sushi mat, or dip your hands in a cold bowl of water and spread the rice with your fingertips, on top layer avocado, cabbage, and slices of cucumber.
3. Using the mat to roll it into a packed roll of rice and vegetable, slide the mat out and repeat.
4. Slice into circles of 1/2 inch. Serve.

Nutrition:
Calories: 135
Total Fat: 3g
Total Carbohydrates: 22g
Fiber: 2g
Sugar: 5g
Protein: 3g

Fascinating Spinach and Beef Meatballs

Preparation time: 10 minutes

Cooking time: 20 minutes

Servings: 4

Ingredients:

- ½ cup onion
- 4 garlic cloves
- 1 whole egg
- ¼ teaspoon oregano
- Pepper as needed
- 1-pound lean ground beef
- 10 ounces spinach

Directions:

1. Preheat your oven to 375 degrees F.
2. Take a bowl and mix in the rest of the ingredients, and using your hands, roll into meatballs.
3. Transfer to a sheet tray and bake for 20 minutes.
4. Enjoy!

Nutrition:

Calorie: 200, Fat: 8g, Carbohydrates: 5g, Protein: 29g

Juicy and Peppery Tenderloin

Preparation time: 10 minutes
Cooking time: 20 minutes
Servings: 4
Ingredients:

- 2 teaspoons sage, chopped
- Sunflower seeds and pepper
- 2 1/2 pounds beef tenderloin
- 2 teaspoons thyme, chopped
- 2 garlic cloves, sliced
- 2 teaspoons rosemary, chopped
- 4 teaspoons olive oil

Directions:

1. Preheat your oven to 425 degrees F.
2. Take a small knife and cut incisions in the tenderloin; insert one slice of garlic into the incision.
3. Rub meat with oil.
4. Take a bowl and add sunflower seeds, sage, thyme, rosemary, pepper and mix well.
5. Rub the spice mix over tenderloin.
6. Put rubbed tenderloin into the roasting pan and bake for 10 minutes.
7. Lower temperature to 350 degrees F and cook for 20 minutes more until an internal thermometer reads 145 degrees F.
8. Transfer tenderloin to a cutting board and let sit for 15 minutes; slice into 20 pieces and enjoy!

Nutrition:
Calorie: 183, Fat: 9g, Carbohydrates: 1g, Protein: 24g

Healthy Avocado Beef Patties

Preparation time: 15 minutes

Cooking time: 10 minutes

Servings: 2

Ingredients:

- 1 pound 85% lean ground beef
- 1 small avocado, pitted and peeled
- Fresh ground black pepper as needed

Directions:

1. Pre-heat and prepare your broiler to high.
2. Divide beef into two equal-sized patties.
3. Season the patties with pepper accordingly.
4. Broil the patties for 5 minutes per side.
5. Transfer the patties to a platter.
6. Slice avocado into strips and place them on top of the patties.
7. Serve and enjoy!

Nutrition:

Calories: 568, Fat: 43g, Net Carbohydrates: 9g, Protein: 38g

Ravaging Beef Pot Roast

Preparation time: 10 minutes

Cooking time: 75 minutes

Servings: 4

Ingredients:

- 3 ½ pounds beef roast
- 4 ounces mushrooms, sliced
- 12 ounces beef stock
- 1-ounce onion soup mix
- ½ cup Italian dressing, low sodium, and low fat

Directions:

1. Take a bowl and add the stock, onion soup mix and Italian dressing.
2. Stir.
3. Put beef roast in pan.
4. Add mushrooms, stock mix to the pan and cover with foil.
5. Preheat your oven to 300 degrees F.
6. Bake for 1 hour and 15 minutes.
7. Let the roast cool. Slice and serve.
8. Enjoy with the gravy on top!

Nutrition:

Calories: 700, Fat: 56g, Carbohydrates: 10g, Protein: 70g

Lovely Faux Mac and Cheese

Preparation time: 15 minutes
Cooking time: 45 minutes
Servings: 4
Ingredients:

- 5 cups cauliflower florets
- Sunflower seeds and pepper to taste
- 1 cup coconut almond milk
- ½ cup vegetable broth
- 2 tablespoons coconut flour, sifted
- 1 organic egg, beaten
- 1 cup cashew cheese

Directions:

1. Preheat your oven to 350 degrees F.
2. Season florets with sunflower seeds and steam until firm.
3. Place florets in a greased ovenproof dish.
4. Heat coconut almond milk over medium heat in a skillet, make sure to season the oil with sunflower seeds and pepper.
5. Stir in broth and add coconut flour to the mix, stir. Cook until the sauce begins to bubble.
6. Remove heat and add beaten egg.
7. Pour the thick sauce over the cauliflower and mix in cheese. Bake for 30-45 minutes.
8. Serve and enjoy!

Nutrition:
Calories: 229; Fat: 14g; Carbohydrates: 9g; Protein: 15g

Epic Mango Chicken

Preparation time: 25 minutes

Cooking time: 10 minutes

Servings: 4

Ingredients:

- 2 medium mangoes, peeled and sliced
- 10-ounce coconut almond milk
- 4 teaspoons vegetable oil
- 4 teaspoons spicy curry paste
- 14-ounce chicken breast halves, skinless and boneless, cut in cubes
- 4 medium shallots
- 1 large English cucumber, sliced and seeded

Directions:

1. Slice half of the mangoes and add the halves to a bowl.
2. Add mangoes and coconut almond milk to a blender and blend until you have a smooth puree.
3. Keep the mixture on the side.
4. Take a large-sized pot and place it over medium heat, add oil and allow the oil to heat up.
5. Add curry paste and cook for 1 minute until you have a nice fragrance, add shallots and chicken to the pot and cook for 5 minutes.
6. Pour mango puree in to the mix and allow it to heat up.
7. Serve the cooked chicken with mango puree and cucumbers.
8. Enjoy!

Nutrition:

Calories: 398; Fat: 20g; Carbohydrates: 32g; Protein: 26g

Chicken and Cabbage Platter

Preparation time: 9 minutes

Cooking time: 14 minutes

Servings: 2

Ingredients:

- ½ cup sliced onion
- 1 tablespoon sesame garlic-flavored oil
- 2 cups shredded Bok-Choy
- 1/2 cups fresh bean sprouts
- 1 1/2 stalks celery, chopped
- 1 ½ teaspoons minced garlic
- 1/2 teaspoon stevia
- 1/2 cup chicken broth
- 1 tablespoon coconut aminos
- 1/2 tablespoon freshly minced ginger
- 1/2 teaspoon arrowroot
- 2 boneless chicken breasts, cooked and sliced thinly

Directions:

1. Shred the cabbage with a knife.
2. Slice onion and add to your platter alongside the rotisserie chicken.
3. Add a dollop of mayonnaise on top and drizzle olive oil over the cabbage.
4. Season with sunflower seeds and pepper according to your taste.
5. Enjoy!

Nutrition:

Calories: 368; Fat: 18g; Net Carbohydrates: 8g; Protein: 42g; Fiber: 3g; Carbohydrates: 11g

Hearty Chicken Liver Stew

Preparation time: 10 minutes
Cooking time: 20 minutes
Servings: 2
Ingredients:

- 10 ounces chicken livers
- 1-ounce onion, chopped
- 2 ounces sour cream
- 1 tablespoon olive oil
- Sunflower seeds to taste

Directions:

1. Take a pan and place it over medium heat.
2. Add oil and let it heat up.
3. Add onions and fry until just browned.
4. Add livers and season with sunflower seeds.
5. Cook until livers are half cooked.
6. Transfer the mix to a stew pot.
7. Add sour cream and cook for 20 minutes.
8. Serve and enjoy!

Nutrition:
Calories: 146; Fat: 9g; Carbohydrates: 2g; Protein: 15g

Chicken Quesadilla

Preparation time: 10 minutes
Cooking time: 35 minutes
Servings: 2
Ingredients:

- ¼ cup ranch dressing
- ½ cup cheddar cheese, shredded
- 20 slices bacon, center-cut
- 2 cups grilled chicken, sliced

Directions:

1. Re-heat your oven to 400 degrees F.
2. Line baking sheet using parchment paper.
3. Weave bacon into two rectangles and bake for 30 minutes.
4. Lay grilled chicken over bacon square, drizzling ranch dressing on top.
5. Sprinkle cheddar cheese and top with another bacon square.
6. Bake for 5 minutes more.
7. Slice and serve.
8. Enjoy!

Nutrition:
Calories: 619, Fat: 35g, Carbohydrates: 2g, Protein: 79g

Mustard Chicken

Preparation time: 10 minutes
Cooking time: 40 minutes
Servings: 2
Ingredients:

- 2 chicken breasts
- 1/4 cup chicken broth
- 2 tablespoons mustard
- 1 1/2 tablespoons olive oil
- 1/2 teaspoon paprika
- 1/2 teaspoon chili powder
- 1/2 teaspoon garlic powder

Directions:

1. Take a small bowl and mix mustard, olive oil, paprika, chicken broth, garlic powder, chicken broth, and chili.
2. Add chicken breast and marinate for 30 minutes.
3. Take a lined baking sheet and arrange the chicken.
4. Bake for 35 minutes at 375 degrees F.
5. Serve and enjoy!

Nutrition:
Calories: 531; Fat: 23g; Carbohydrates: 10g; Protein: 64g

Chicken and Carrot Stew

Preparation time: 15 minutes
Cooking time: 6 minutes
Servings: 4
Ingredients:

- 4 boneless chicken breasts, cubed
- 3 cups of carrots, peeled and cubed
- 1 cup onion, chopped
- 1 cup tomatoes, chopped
- 1 teaspoon of dried thyme
- 2 cups of chicken broth
- 2 garlic cloves, minced
- Sunflower seeds and pepper as needed

Directions:

1. Add all of the listed ingredients to a Slow Cooker.
2. Stir and close the lid.
3. Cook for 6 hours.
4. Serve hot and enjoy!

Nutrition:
Calories: 182, Fat: 3g, Carbohydrates: 10g, Protein: 39g

The Delish Turkey Wrap

Preparation time: 10 minutes

Cooking time: 10 minutes

Servings: 6

Ingredients:

- 1 ¼ pounds ground turkey, lean
- 4 green onions, minced
- 1 tablespoon olive oil
- 1 garlic clove, minced
- 2 teaspoons chili paste
- 8-ounce water chestnut, diced
- 3 tablespoons hoisin sauce
- 2 tablespoon coconut aminos
- 1 tablespoon rice vinegar
- 12 almond butter lettuce leaves
- 1/8 teaspoon sunflower seeds

Directions:

1. Take a pan and place it over medium heat, add turkey and garlic to the pan.
2. Heat for 6 minutes until cooked.
3. Take a bowl and transfer turkey to the bowl.
4. Add onions and water chestnuts.
5. Stir in hoisin sauce, coconut aminos, and vinegar and chili paste.
6. Toss well and transfer mix to lettuce leaves.
7. Serve and enjoy!

Nutrition:

Calories: 162; Fat: 4g; Net Carbohydrates: 7g; Protein: 23g

Almond butternut Chicken

Preparation time: 15 minutes
Cooking time: 30 minutes
Servings: 4
Ingredients:

- ½ pound Nitrate free bacon
- 6 chicken thighs, boneless and skinless
- 2-3 cups almond butternut squash, cubed
- Extra virgin olive oil
- Fresh chopped sage
- Sunflower seeds and pepper as needed

Directions:

1. Prepare your oven by preheating it to 425 degrees F.
2. Take a large skillet and place it over medium-high heat, add bacon and fry until crispy.
3. Take a slice of bacon and place it on the side, crumble the bacon.
4. Add cubed almond butternut squash in the bacon grease and sauté, season with sunflower seeds and pepper.
5. Once the squash is tender, remove skillet and transfer to a plate.
6. Add coconut oil to the skillet and add chicken thighs, cook for 10 minutes.
7. Season with sunflower seeds and pepper.
8. Remove skillet from stove and transfer to oven.
9. Bake for 12-15 minutes, top with the crumbled bacon and sage.
10.   Enjoy!

Nutrition:
Calories: 323; Fat: 19g; Carbohydrates: 8g; Protein: 12g

Zucchini Zoodles with Chicken and Basil

Preparation time: 10 minutes
Cooking time: 10 minutes
Servings: 3
Ingredients:

- 2 chicken fillets, cubed
- 2 tablespoons ghee
- 1-pound tomatoes, diced
- ½ cup basil, chopped
- ¼ cup almond milk
- 1 garlic clove, peeled, minced
- 1 zucchini, shredded

Directions:

1. Sauté cubed chicken in ghee until no longer pink.
2. Add tomatoes and season with sunflower seeds.
3. Simmer and reduce liquid.
4. Prepare your zucchini Zoodles by shredding zucchini in a food processor.
5. Add basil, garlic, coconut almond milk to the chicken and cook for a few minutes.
6. Add half of the zucchini Zoodles to a bowl and top with creamy tomato basil chicken.
7. Enjoy!

Nutrition:
Calories: 540; Fat: 27g; Carbohydrates: 13g; Protein: 59g

Duck with Cucumber and Carrots

Preparation time: 10 minutes

Cooking time: 40 minutes

Servings: 8

Ingredients:

- 1 duck, cut up into medium pieces
- 1 chopped cucumber, chopped
- 1 tablespoon low sodium vegetable stock
- 2 carrots, chopped
- 2 cups of water
- Black pepper as needed
- 1-inch ginger piece, grated

Directions:

1. Add duck pieces to your Instant Pot.
2. Add cucumber, stock, carrots, water, ginger, pepper and stir.
3. Lock up the lid and cook on LOW pressure for 40 minutes.
4. Release the pressure naturally.
5. Serve and enjoy!

Nutrition:

Calories: 206; Fats: 7g; Carbs: 28g; Protein: 16g

Parmesan Baked Chicken

Preparation time: 5 minutes
Cooking time: 20 minutes
Servings: 2
Ingredients:

- 2 tablespoons ghee
- 2 boneless chicken breasts, skinless
- Pink sunflower seeds
- Freshly ground black pepper
- ½ cup mayonnaise, low fat
- ¼ cup parmesan cheese, grated
- 1 tablespoon dried Italian seasoning, low fat, low sodium
- ¼ cup crushed pork rinds

Directions:

1. Preheat your oven to 425 degrees F.
2. Take a large baking dish and coat with ghee.
3. Pat chicken breasts dry and wrap with a towel.
4. Season with sunflower seeds and pepper.
5. Place in baking dish.
6. Take a small bowl and add mayonnaise, parmesan cheese, Italian seasoning.
7. Slather mayo mix evenly over chicken breast.
8. Sprinkle crushed pork rinds on top.
9. Bake for 20 minutes until topping is browned.
10. Serve and enjoy!

Nutrition:
Calories: 850; Fat: 67g; Carbohydrates: 2g; Protein: 60g

Buffalo Chicken Lettuce Wraps

Preparation time: 35 minutes
Cooking time: 10 minutes
Servings: 2
Ingredients:
- 3 chicken breasts, boneless and cubed
- 20 slices of almond butter lettuce leaves
- ¾ cup cherry tomatoes halved
- 1 avocado, chopped
- ¼ cup green onions, diced
- ½ cup ranch dressing
- ¾ cup hot sauce

Directions:

1. Take a mixing bowl and add chicken cubes and hot sauce, mix.
2. Place in the fridge and let it marinate for 30 minutes.
3. Preheat your oven to 400 degrees F.
4. Place coated chicken on a cookie pan and bake for 9 minutes.
5. Assemble lettuce serving cups with equal amounts of lettuce, green onions, tomatoes, ranch dressing, and cubed chicken.
6. Serve and enjoy!

Nutrition:

Calories: 106; Fat: 6g; Net Carbohydrates: 2g; Protein: 5g

Crazy Japanese Potato and Beef Croquettes

Preparation time: 10 minutes

Cooking time: 20 minutes

Servings: 10

Ingredients:

- 3 medium russet potatoes, peeled and chopped
- 1 tablespoon almond butter
- 1 tablespoon vegetable oil
- 3 onions, diced
- ¾ pound ground beef
- 4 teaspoons light coconut aminos
- All-purpose flour for coating
- 2 eggs, beaten
- Panko bread crumbs for coating
- ½ cup oil, frying

Directions:

1. Take a saucepan and place it over medium-high heat; add potatoes and sunflower seeds water, boil for 16 minutes.
2. Remove water and put potatoes in another bowl, add almond butter and mash the potatoes.
3. Take a frying pan and place it over medium heat, add 1 tablespoon oil and let it heat up.
4. Add onions and stir fry until tender.
5. Add coconut aminos to beef to onions.
6. Keep frying until beef is browned.
7. Mix the beef with the potatoes evenly.
8. Take another frying pan and place it over medium heat; add half a cup of oil.
9. Form croquettes using the mashed potato mixture and coat them with flour, then eggs and finally breadcrumbs.
10. Fry patties until golden on all sides.
11. Enjoy!

Nutrition:

Calories: 239; Fat: 4g; Carbohydrates: 20g; Protein: 10g

Spicy Chili Crackers

Preparation time: 15 minutes
Cooking time: 60 minutes
Servings: 30 crackers
Ingredients:

- ¾ cup almond flour
- ¼ cup coconut four
- ¼ cup coconut flour
- ½ teaspoon paprika
- ½ teaspoon cumin
- 1 ½ teaspoons chili pepper spice
- 1 teaspoon onion powder
- ½ teaspoon sunflower seeds
- 1 whole egg
- ¼ cup unsalted almond butter

Directions:

1. Preheat your oven to 350 degrees F.
2. Line a baking sheet with parchment paper and keep it on the side.
3. Add ingredients to your food processor and pulse until you have a nice dough.
4. Divide dough into two equal parts.
5. Place one ball on a sheet of parchment paper and cover with another sheet; roll it out.
6. Cut into crackers and repeat with the other ball.
7. Transfer the prepped dough to a baking tray and bake for 8-10 minutes.
8. Remove from oven and serve.
9. Enjoy!

Nutrition:
Total Carbs: 2.8g, Fiber: 1, Protein: 1.6g, Fat: 4.1g

Golden Eggplant Fries

Preparation time: 10 minutes
Cooking time: 15 minutes
Servings: 8
Ingredients:
- 2 eggs
- 2 cups almond flour
- 2 tablespoons coconut oil, spray
- 2 eggplant, peeled and cut thinly
- Sunflower seeds and pepper

Directions:
1. Preheat your oven to 400 degrees F.
2. Take a bowl and mix with sunflower seeds and black pepper.
3. Take another bowl and beat eggs until frothy.
4. Dip the eggplant pieces into the eggs.
5. Then coat them with the flour mixture.
6. Add another layer of flour and egg.
7. Then, take a baking sheet and grease with coconut oil on top.
8. Bake for about 15 minutes.
9. Serve and enjoy!

Nutrition:
Calories: 212, Fat: 15.8g, Carbohydrates: 12.1g, Protein: 8.6g

CHAPTER 6:

Dinner

Turkey Stir Fry with Vegetables

Preparation Time: 10 minutes
Cooking Time: 30 minutes
Servings: 2
Ingredients:
- 1 Cup turkey, cooked, cut into 1/2-inch cubes
- 2 Cups vegetables, fresh or frozen or canned
- 2 cups brown rice, cooked
- 1 Tablespoon oil
- 1/2 teaspoon sugar
- 1/2 Tablespoon ginger, minced
- 1/4 Teaspoon clove Garlic, minced
- 1/2 teaspoon salt

Directions:
1. In a non-stick frying pan, heat oil at low-medium temperature.
2. Put the turkey, vegetables, minced ginger, garlic, and salt.
3. Stir and fry for about one minute.
4. Add sugar and continue stirring.
5. Reduce heat to avoid scorching and continue cooking until the vegetables become tender.
6. When the vegetables become tender, remove them from the heat.
7. In the event, if the vegetables did not cook well, pour 2-3 tablespoons of water and cook until it becomes soft.
8. Serve with the cooked rice.

Nutrition:
Calories: 223
Total Fat: 12g
Total Carbohydrates: 21g
Fiber: 6g
Sugar: 8g
Protein: 13g

Tuscan White Beans with Shrimp, Spinach, and Feta

Preparation Time: 10 minutes

Cooking Time: 20 minutes

Servings: 2

Ingredients:

1 Pound shrimp, large, peeled, and deveined

15 Ounces cannellini beans, saltless, rinsed and drained

1 1/2 Ounces low-fat feta cheese, shredded

1/2 cup chicken broth, fat-free, low-sodium

4 Cloves clove Garlic, minced

2 Teaspoons sage, fresh, finely chopped

2 Tablespoons balsamic vinegar

2 Tablespoons olive oil

1 medium-size onion, chopped

5 cups baby spinach

Directions:

1. Take a large skillet
2. Pour one tablespoon of olive oil and bring to medium temperature.
3. When the oil becomes hot, put the shrimp for 2-3 minutes.
4. Transfer the shrimp to a plate when its color changes.
5. Pour the balance oil into the skillet and put chopped onion, sage, and garlic.
6. Stir and cook until the onion turns a golden color. Within 4 minutes of cooking, the onion will start to become a golden color.
7. Add vinegar and continue cooking for another half minute.
8. Now add the chicken broth and cook for two minutes until it boils.
9. At this time, add the vegetables and put the spinach. Cook until the spinach starts to wilt.
10. Get the skillet from the heat and put the cooked shrimp and stir.
11. Serve by topping with feta cheese.

Nutrition:

Calories: 280

Total Fat: 7g

Total Carbohydrates: 22g

Fiber: 6g

Sugar: 0.5g
Protein: 32g

Chicken & Broccoli in Sesame Noodles

Preparation Time: 5 minutes
Cooking Time: 20 minutes
Servings: 2
Ingredients:
- 1/2 Cup chicken, cooked & diced
- 8 Ounces whole-wheat spaghetti noodles
- 1/4 cup vegetable oil
- 12 Ounces broccoli florets, frozen
- 1 Tablespoon garlic, minced
- 2 Tablespoons sugar
- 2 Tablespoons rice vinegar
- 2 Tablespoons soy sauce, low sodium
- 1 Tablespoon sesame seeds, toasted

Directions:
1. Prepare pasta as per the package instructions and keep it aside.
2. In a medium bowl, whisk soy sauce, sugar, and vinegar and keep aside.
3. Add the oil in a skillet and bring to medium heat.
4. Put broccoli and garlic and cook until it becomes soft.
5. Now add the chicken pieces and cook very well for about 10 minutes.
6. When the chicken's color starts to change, add soy sauce mixture and pasta.
7. Mix it thoroughly.
8. Serve by drizzling sesame seeds on top.

Nutrition:
Calories: 240
Total Fat: 9g
Total Carbohydrates: 27g
Fiber: 4g
Sugar: 5g
Protein: 13g

Spicy Baked Potatoes

Preparation Time: 10 minutes

Cooking Time: 25 minutes

Servings: 2

Ingredients:

- 4 medium-size sweet potatoes
- 1/3 cups black beans, canned, rinsed and drained
- 1/2 cup Greek yogurt no-fat
- 1 Teaspoon olive oil
- 1 Teaspoon taco seasoning, low sodium
- 1/2 cup red pepper, diced
- 1/2 cup onion, chopped
- 1/2 teaspoon paprika
- 1 teaspoon chili powder
- 1/2 Teaspoon cumin
- 1/2 cup Mexican cheese, low-fat
- 1/4 teaspoon salt
- 1/2 cup salsa

Directions:

1. Make holes in the potato with a fork or any sharp kitchen tools.
2. Microwave it for about 8-10 minutes until it becomes tender.
3. In a bowl, mix taco seasoning with yogurt.
4. Now heat oil in a saucepan at medium temperature.
5. Put chopped onions, paprika, chili powder, peppers, cumin, and sauté continuously on medium heat until the onion gets caramelized.
6. Add salt and continue stirring. Wait for about 5 minutes to get the onion caramelized.
7. Now add the drained black beans; continue heating and stirring for about 5 minutes.
8. Using a fork, slice the potato lengthwise.
9. Serve it by dressing with 2 tablespoons of shredded cheese, 2 tablespoons of Greek yogurt mixture, black bean mixture 1/3, and 2 tablespoons of salsa.

Nutrition:

Calories: 260

Total Fat: 15g

Total Carbohydrates: 32g
Fiber: 6g
Sugar: 3g
Protein: 5g

Tandoori Chicken

Preparation Time: 10 minutes

Cooking Time: 20 minutes

Servings: 2

Ingredients:

- 6 Pieces boneless chicken cut into 1-inch pieces
- 1 cup yogurt, plain, fatless
- 2 Tablespoons paprika
- 1 teaspoon yellow curry powder
- 1 teaspoon red pepper, crushed
- 1/2 cup lemon juice
- 5 cloves garlic cloves, minced
- 1 teaspoon ground ginger
- 6 Skewers, soaked in water for 15 minutes

Directions:

1. Using a blender, combine yogurt, garlic, lemon juice, curry powder, red pepper, ginger, and paprika thoroughly until it becomes a smooth paste.
2. Set your over to 390°F and preheat.
3. On the soaked skewers, skew all chicken pieces.
4. Place the skewed chicken on a plain plate and marinate the chicken with the blended mix. Keep the remaining marinade mix for later use.
5. Cover the marinated skewed chicken and refrigerate for a better marinade effect.
6. Let it marinates for about 4 hours and after that, take it out and again brush with the remaining marinade mix.
7. Now, bake it for about 20 minutes or bake it until the chicken's secretion from the chicken stops or the meat gets pierced. Serve hot.

Nutrition:

Calories: 112

Total Fat: 2g

Total Carbohydrates: 11g

Fiber: 2g

Sugar: 1g

Protein: 10g

Pork Tenderloin with Sweet Potatoes & Apple

Preparation Time: 10 minutes
Cooking Time: 30 minutes
Servings: 2
Ingredients:
- 12 Ounces of pork tenderloin
- 1 Potato, large, cut into 1/2" cubes
- 3/4 cup apple cider
- 1/4 cup apple cider vinegar
- 1/4 Teaspoon paprika, smoked
- 2 Tablespoons maple syrup
- 1/4 Teaspoon ginger, dried
- 1 Teaspoon ginger, fresh, minced
- 2 Tablespoons vegetable oil
- 1 Apple, cut into 1/2" cube size

Directions:
1. Take a large bowl and start mixing smoked paprika, apple cider, maple syrup, apple cider vinegar, black pepper, ginger, and keep aside.
2. Set your oven to 360°F and preheat.
3. Take a large oven-safe sauté pan and heat oil at medium temperature.
4. Once the oil becomes hot, put the pork tenderloin. Continue cooking at medium temperature for about 10 minutes.
5. Flip sides and make sure to cook all sides evenly. Once the sides cooked well, remove them from the heat.
6. Arrange the sweet potatoes around the tenderloin. Pour apple cider mixture over it.
7. Cover the saucepan and bake it for about 10 minutes.
8. Place the sliced apple pieces around the pork tenderloin and bake for another 10 minutes, until the tenderloin temperature shows 340°F.
9. Once the temperature is reached at 340°F, stop baking and remove the pork tenderloin, potatoes and apple and allow it to settle for 10 minutes.
10. Heat the cider mixture and reduce to 1/4 cup.
11. Slice the pork to edible size. Serve along with sweet potatoes and apples.

12.   Dress it with apple cider while serving.

Nutrition:

Calories: 339

Total Fat: 12g

Total Carbohydrates: 21g

Fiber: 3g

Sugar: 0g

Protein: 35g

Tasty Tortilla Bake

Preparation Time: 15 minutes
Cooking Time: 30 minutes
Servings: 2
Ingredients:

- 8 Tortilla, sliced into half
- 1 cup corn, frozen or fresh
- 1 Onion, green, chopped
- 3 Eggs
- 1 cup milk, fat-free
- 1 cup Monterey Jack cheese
- 1 cup black beans, cooked
- 2 Ounces green chilies, canned, chopped
- 1/2 teaspoon chili powder
- 1 Tomato, sliced
- 1/4 teaspoon salsa

Directions:

1. Take an 8" square shaped baking tray and spray some cooking oil.
2. Set your oven to 370°F and preheat.
3. Layer in 5 tortilla halves in the bottom of the baking pan.
4. Top it with one-third of the cheese, beans, and corn layer by layer. Repeat the layering.
5. Beat egg in a bowl with chili powder, green chili, and milk. Now pour the mix over the tortilla.
6. Dress the tomato slice over the tortilla and spread the remaining cheese on top.
7. Bake it for 30 minutes and check to confirm its baking status.
8. Allow it to settle for another 10 minutes.
9. Serve with salsa.

Nutrition:
Calories: 181
Total Fat: 8g
Total Carbohydrates: 21g
Fiber: 0g
Sugar: 4g
Protein: 4g

Pear Quesadillas

Preparation Time: 10 minutes
Cooking Time: 15 minutes
Servings: 2
Ingredients:

- 1 Cup pear, canned or fresh, cubed
- 1 cup cheddar cheese, grated
- 4 Medium size whole-wheat tortillas
- 1/2 cup green peppers, thinly chopped
- 2 Tablespoons Onion, finely chopped

Directions:

1. Place two tortillas on a cutting board.
2. Drizzle 1/4 of the shredded cheese on both tortillas.
3. Equally divide the peppers, pears, and onion and place on both tortillas. Now place the remaining cheese on both tortillas.
4. Top the tortillas with the remaining two tortillas.
5. Take large non-stick sauté pan and bring to medium heat. Place the tortillas in the pan.
6. Cook for about 3-4 minutes until the bottoms side becomes slightly brown.
7. Using a spatula, flip the tortilla and cook the other side for 3-4 minutes.
8. Once it is ready, gently transfer to a serving plate and cook the second tortillas.
9. Follow the same preceding Directions and cook until it is ready.
10. Before serving, cut the tortillas into 4 eatable sizes.
11. Serve hot, and you can refrigerate the balance for later consumption.

Nutrition:
Calories: 217
Total Fat: 11g
Total Carbohydrates: 19g
Fiber: 2g
Sugar: 5g
Protein: 10g

Porcini Mushrooms with Pasta

Preparation Time: 15 minutes
Cooking Time: 20 minutes
Servings: 2
Ingredients:
- 1/4 Ounce porcini mushrooms, dried
- 1/2 Tablespoon onion, thinly chopped
- 3 Tablespoons tomatoes, sun-dried, drained, sliced
- 1/2 cup evaporated skim milk
- 1/8 Teaspoon pepper, white, grounded
- 1/2 Pound pasta
- 1 Green onion, cut into 1/4" diagonal shape
- 1 Tablespoon parmesan cheese, grated
- 1 Teaspoon butter, unsalted
- 1/8 Teaspoon salt

Directions:
1. Wash mushrooms in running water. Put it in a hot water bowl for 10 minutes.
2. After that, drain and slice the mushrooms into 1/2" size.
3. Take a large non-stick sauté pan, put butter, and heat on medium temperature.
4. When the butter melted, add shallots and sauté for about one minute.
5. Now, add tomatoes and mushrooms and stir for about three minutes.
6. Pour milk, white pepper ground, salt, and bring to boil.
7. Wait for 15 minutes to simmer and let the volume reduce to a quarter.
8. Now cook the pasta in hot water. Once the pasta is cooked well, drain the water and shift the pasta to a serving bowl.
9. Transfer the sauce over the pasta and toss to mix it properly.
10. Drizzle the shredded parmesan cheese and scallions while serving.

Nutrition:
Calories: 200
Total Fat: 2g
Total Carbohydrates: 39g
Fiber: 2g

Sugar: 0g
Protein: 8g

Shrimp & Nectarine Salad

Preparation Time: 10 minutes

Cooking Time: 20 minutes

Servings: 2

Ingredients:

- 1/3 cup orange juice
- 3 tablespoons cider vinegar
- 1-1/2 teaspoons Dijon mustard
- 1-1/2 teaspoons honey
- 1 tablespoon minced fresh tarragon

Salad:

- 4 teaspoons canola oil, divided
- 1 cup fresh or frozen corn
- 1-pound shrimp, uncooked, peeled and deveined
- 1/2 teaspoon lemon-pepper seasoning
- 1/4 teaspoon salt
- 8 cups torn mixed salad greens
- 1 medium nectarines, cut into 1-inch pieces
- 1 cup grape tomatoes, halved
- 1/2 cup finely chopped red onion

Directions:

1. Mix orange juice, vinegar, mustard, and honey in a bowl until blended. Stir in tarragon.
2. With a medium skillet, heat 1 tsp oil over medium-high heat. Input your corn; keep cooking and stirring until 1-2 minutes or until crisp-soft. Keep away from the pan.
3. Spray shrimp with lemon, pepper, and salt. With the same skillet, heat leftover oil over medium-high heat. Put together shrimp; cook and stir 3-4 minutes or till you see shrimp turn pink. Stir in corn.
4. With a large pan, combine leftover ingredients. Drizzle with 1/3 cup dressing and toss to coat it.
5. Separate the mixture among four plates. Add with shrimp mixture; drizzle with leftover dressing. Serve warm.

Nutrition:

Calories: 250

Total Fat: 7g

Total Carbohydrates: 27g
Fiber: 5g
Sugar: 10g
Protein: 23g

Pork Chops with Tomato Curry

Preparation Time: 15 minutes
Cooking Time: 25 minutes
Servings: 2
Ingredients:

- 6 pork loin chops, boneless (6 oz. each)
- 1 small onion
- 4 teaspoons butter (divided)
- 2 medium apples, sliced thinly
- 1 can whole tomatoes, undrained
- 2 teaspoons sugar
- 2 teaspoons curry powder
- 1/2 teaspoon salt
- 1/2 teaspoon chili powder
- 2 cups hot cooked brown rice
- 2 tablespoons toasted slivered almonds, optional

Directions:

1. Finely chopped the onion.
2. Prepare a stockpot, warm 2 teaspoons butter over medium-high heat. Brown pork chops in batches. Remove from pan.
3. Warm remaining butter in the same pan with over medium heat. Include onions; keep cooking and stirring 2-3 minutes or until softened.
4. Keep turning the apples, tomatoes, sugar, curry powder, salt, and chili powder. Gather to a boil, stirring consciously to break up tomatoes.
5. Return chops to pan. Reduce heat; simmer, uncovered, 5 minutes. Keep turning chops; cook it up to 3-5 minutes longer or until a thermometer inserted in pork are reads 145°.
6. Allow it cool for 5 minutes' minimum before serving. Serve with rice and, if desired, sprinkle with almonds.

Nutrition:
Calories: 143 Total Fat: 6g
Total Carbohydrates: 9g Fiber: 2g
Sugar: 6g Protein: 12g

Thai Chicken Pasta Skillet

Preparation Time: 10 minutes
Cooking Time: 20 minutes
Servings: 2
Ingredients:
- 6 ounces uncooked whole-wheat spaghetti
- 2 tsp. canola oil
- 1 package fresh sugar snap peas, trimmed and cut diagonally into thin strips
- 2 cups julienned carrots (about 8 ounces)
- 2 cups shredded cooked chicken
- 1 cup Thai peanut sauce
- 1 medium cucumber, halved lengthwise, seeded, and sliced diagonally
- Chopped fresh cilantro, optional

Directions:
1. Cook pasta consistent with package Directions, drain.
2. Meanwhile, in a frying pan, warm oil over medium-high heat. Add snap peas and carrots; stir-fry 6-8 minutes or till crisp tender.
3. Add chicken, peanut sauce, and spaghetti; heat through, moving to mix.
4. Transfer to a serving plate. Add cucumber and, if desired, cilantro.

Nutrition:
Calories: 400 Total Fat: 15g
Total Carbohydrates: 40g
Fiber: 6g Sugar: 10g Protein: 25g

Chili-Lime Grilled Pineapple

Preparation Time: 5 minutes
Cooking Time: 10 minutes
Servings: 2
Ingredients:

- 1 fresh pineapple
- 2 tablespoons brown sugar
- 2 tablespoon lime juice
- 1 tablespoon olive oil
- 1 tablespoon honey or agave nectar
- 1-1/2 teaspoons chili powder
- Dash salt

Directions:

1. Peel pineapple, removing any eyes from fruit.
2. Cut lengthwise into wedges; take away the core. In a very little bowl, combine the remaining ingredients till blended.
3. Brush pineapple with half the glaze; reserve the remaining mixture for basting.
4. Grill pineapple, for 2-4 minutes on each side or until lightly browned, occasionally basting with reserved glaze.

Nutrition:
Calories: 97 Total Fat: 2g
Total Carbohydrates: 20g
Fiber: 1g Sugar: 17g
Proteins: 1g

Peppered Sole

Preparation Time: 10 minutes
Cooking Time: 15 minutes
Servings: 2
Ingredients:
- 2 tablespoons butter
- 2 cups sliced fresh mushrooms
- 2 garlic cloves, minced
- 4 sole fillets (4 ounces each)
- 1/4 teaspoon paprika
- 1/4 teaspoon lemon-pepper seasoning
- 1/8 teaspoon cayenne pepper
- 1 medium tomato, chopped
- 1 green onions, thinly sliced

Directions:
1. Using a large skillet, heat butter over medium-high heat. Put mushrooms; cook and stir until softened.
2. Put garlic; cook 1 minute longer. Place fillets over mushrooms. Sprinkle with paprika, lemon pepper, and cayenne.
3. Cover and cook it over medium heat 5-10 minutes or until fish begins to flake easily with a fork.
4. Sprinkle with tomato and green onions.

Nutrition:
Calories: 25
Total Fat: 16g
Total Carbohydrates: 18g
Fiber: 0g
Sugar: 2g
Protein: 10g

Shrimp Orzo with Feta

Preparation Time: 10 minutes
Cooking Time: 15 minutes
Servings: 2
Ingredients:

- 1-1/4 cups whole wheat orzo pasta (uncooked)
- 2 tbsp. olive oil
- 2 garlic cloves
- 2 medium tomatoes
- 2 tbsp. lemon juice
- 1-1/4 lb. uncooked shrimp (peeled and deveined)
- 2 tbsp. minced fresh cilantro
- 1/4 tsp. pepper
- 1/2 cup feta cheese (crumbled)

Directions:

1. Chopped 2 medium tomatoes and 2 garlic cloves.
2. Cook orzo according to package Directions. Better still, in a large pan, heat oil over a medium cooker.
3. Put garlic; cook and stir 1 minute. Include tomatoes and lemon juice. Then to a boil. Stir in shrimp.
4. Decrease the heat; simmer and uncover it until shrimp turn pink, 4-5 minutes.
5. Dry orzo, cilantro, and pepper to shrimp together; heat through.
6. Spray with feta cheese.

Nutrition:
Calories: 340
Total Fat: 14g
Total Carbohydrates: 33g
Fiber: 4g
Sugar: 2g
Protein: 22g

Beef and Blue Cheese Penne with Pesto

Preparation Time: 15 minutes

Cooking Time: 15 minutes

Servings: 2

Ingredients:

- 2 cups uncooked whole wheat penne pasta
- 2 beef tenderloin steaks (6 ounces each)
- 1/4 teaspoon salt
- 1/4 teaspoon pepper
- 5 oz. fresh baby spinach (about 6 cups), coarsely chopped
- 2 cups grape tomatoes, halved
- 1/3 cup prepared pesto
- 1/4 cup chopped walnuts
- 1/4 cup crumbled Gorgonzola cheese

Directions:

1. Cook pasta according to package Directions.
2. . Meanwhile, sprinkle steaks with salt and pepper for under 5-7 minutes on each side or until meat reaches desired doneness. For medium thermometer should read 135°F; medium, 140°F; medium-well, 145°F).
3. Drain pasta; transfer to a large bowl. Add spinach, tomatoes, pesto, and walnuts; toss to coat.
4. Cut steak into thin slices. Serve pasta mixture with beef; sprinkle with cheese.

Nutrition:

Calories: 530

Total Fat: 20g

Total Carbohydrates: 49g

Fiber: 9g

Sugar: 0g

Protein: 35g

California Quinoa

Preparation Time: 10 minutes
Cooking Time: 20 minutes
Servings: 2
Ingredients:
- 1 tablespoon olive oil
- 1 cup quinoa, rinsed and well-drained
- 2 garlic cloves, minced
- 1 medium zucchini, chopped
- 2 cups of water
- 3/4 cup garbanzo beans or chickpeas (canned)
- 1 medium tomato, finely chopped
- 1/2 cup crumbled feta cheese
- 1/4 cup finely chopped Greek olives
- 2 tablespoons minced fresh basil
- 1/4 teaspoon pepper

Directions:
1. Rinsed and drained garbanzo beans or chickpeas.
2. With a large saucepan, heat oil across medium heat.
3. Include quinoa and garlic; stir and cook until 2-3 minutes or until quinoa is lightly colored.
4. Stir together in zucchini and water; bring to heat. Decrease to heat; simmer, covered, till liquid is dry, 12-15 minutes.
5. Stir in the leftover ingredients; heat thoroughly.

Nutrition:
Calories: 160
Total Fat: 7g
Total Carbohydrates: 20g
Fiber: 4g
Sugar: 10g
Protein: 4g

Peppered Tuna Kabobs

Preparation Time: 10 minutes
Cooking Time: 20 minutes
Servings:
Ingredients:

- 1/2 cup frozen corn, thawed
- 4 green onions
- 1 jalapeno pepper, seeded
- 2 tablespoons fresh parsley
- 1 tbsp. lime juice
- 1 lb. tuna steaks, cut into 1-inch cubes
- 1 tsp. coarsely ground pepper
- 1 medium mango, peeled
- 2 large sweet red peppers

Directions:

1. Chopped green onions, fresh parsley and jalapeno pepper.
2. Cut mango into 1-inch cubes and red peppers into 2x1 inch.
3. Add salsa, in a little bowl, add the first five ingredients; set aside.
4. Rub tuna with pepper. Use four metal or soaked wooden skewers or thread red peppers, tuna, and mango.
5. Use skewers on a greased grill rack. Cover it and cook over medium heat, keep always turning, until tuna is slightly turned to pink in center (medium-rare) and peppers are soft, 10-12 minutes.
6. Good with salsa.

Nutrition:
Calories: 205
Total Fat: 2g
Total Carbohydrates: 20g
Fiber: 4g
Sugar: 12g
Protein: 29g

Shrimp Cocktail

Preparation time: 10 minutes
Cooking time: 5 minutes
Servings: 8
Ingredients:

- 2 pounds big shrimp, deveined
- 4 cups of water
- 2 bay leaves
- 1 small lemon, halved
- Ice for cooling the shrimp
- Ice for serving
- 1 medium lemon sliced for serving
- ¾ cup tomato passata
- 2 and ½ tablespoons horseradish, prepared
- ¼ teaspoon chili powder
- 2 tablespoons lemon juice

Directions:

1. Pour the 4 cups water into a large pot, add lemon and bay leaves. Boil over medium-high heat, reduce temperature, and boil for 10 minutes. Put shrimp, stir and cook within 2 minutes. Move the shrimp to a bowl filled with ice and leave aside for 5 minutes.
2. In a bowl, mix tomato passata with horseradish, chili powder, and lemon juice and stir well.
3. Place shrimp in a serving bowl filled with ice, with lemon slices, and serve with the cocktail sauce you've prepared.

Nutrition:
Calories: 276; Carbs: 0g; Fat: 8g; Protein: 25g; Sodium: 182 mg

Quinoa and Scallops Salad

Preparation time: 10 minutes
Cooking time: 35 minutes
Servings: 6
Ingredients:
- 12 ounces dry sea scallops
- 4 tablespoons canola oil
- 2 teaspoons canola oil
- 4 teaspoons low sodium soy sauce
- 1 and ½ cup quinoa, rinsed
- 2 teaspoons garlic, minced
- 3 cups of water
- 1 cup snow peas, sliced diagonally
- 1 teaspoon sesame oil
- 1/3 cup rice vinegar
- 1 cup scallions, sliced
- 1/3 cup red bell pepper, chopped
- ¼ cup cilantro, chopped

Directions:
1. In a bowl, mix scallops with 2 teaspoons soy sauce, stir gently, and leave aside for now. Heat a pan with 1 tablespoon canola oil over medium-high heat, add the quinoa, stir and cook for 8 minutes. Put garlic, stir and cook within 1 more minute.
2. Put the water, boil over medium heat, stir, cover, and cook for 15 minutes. Remove from heat and leave aside covered for 5 minutes. Add snow peas, cover again and leave for 5 more minutes.
3. Meanwhile, in a bowl, mix 3 tablespoons canola oil with 2 teaspoons soy sauce, vinegar, and sesame oil and stir well. Add quinoa and snow peas to this mixture and stir again. Add scallions, bell pepper, and stir again.
4. Pat dry the scallops and discard marinade. Heat another pan with 2 teaspoons canola oil over high heat, add scallops, and cook for 1 minute on each side. Add them to the quinoa salad, stir gently, and serve with chopped cilantro.

Nutrition:

Calories: 181; Carbs: 12g; Fat: 6g; Protein: 13g; Sodium: 153 mg

Squid and Shrimp Salad

Preparation time: 10 minutes

Cooking time: 15 minutes

Servings: 4

Ingredients:

- 8 ounces squid, cut into medium pieces
- 8 ounces shrimp, peeled and deveined
- 1 red onion, sliced
- 1 cucumber, chopped
- 2 tomatoes, cut into medium wedges
- 2 tablespoons cilantro, chopped
- 1 hot jalapeno pepper, cut in rounds
- 3 tablespoons rice vinegar
- 3 tablespoons dark sesame oil
- Black pepper to the taste

Directions:

1. In a bowl, mix the onion with cucumber, tomatoes, pepper, cilantro, shrimp, and squid and stir well. Cut a big parchment paper in half, fold it in half heart shape and open. Place the seafood mixture in this parchment piece, fold over, seal edges, place on a baking sheet, and introduce in the oven at 400 degrees F for 15 minutes.
2. Meanwhile, in a small bowl, mix sesame oil with rice vinegar and black pepper and stir very well. Take the salad out of the oven, leave to cool down for a few minutes, and transfer to a serving plate.

3. Put the dressing over the salad and serve right away.
Nutrition:
Calories: 235; Carbs: 9g; Fat: 8g; Protein: 30g; Sodium: 165 mg

Parsley Seafood Cocktail

Preparation time: 2 hours and 10 minutes
Cooking time: 1 hour and 30 minutes
Servings: 4
Ingredients:

- 1 big octopus, cleaned
- 1-pound mussels
- 2 pounds clams
- 1 big squid cut in rings
- 3 garlic cloves, chopped
- 1 celery rib, cut crosswise into thirds
- ½ cup celery rib, sliced
- 1 carrot, cut crosswise into 3 pieces
- 1 small white onion, chopped
- 1 bay leaf
- ¾ cup white wine
- 2 cups radicchio, sliced
- 1 red onion, sliced
- 1 cup parsley, chopped
- 1 cup olive oil
- 1 cup red wine vinegar
- Black pepper to the taste

Directions:

1. Put the octopus in a pot with celery rib cut in thirds, garlic, carrot, bay leaf, white onion, and white wine. Add water to cover the octopus, cover with a lid, bring to a boil over high heat, reduce to low, and simmer within 1 and ½ hours.

2. Drain octopus, reserve boiling liquid, and leave aside to cool down. Put ¼ cup octopus cooking liquid in another pot, add mussels, and heat up over medium-high heat, cook until they open, transfer to a bowl, and leave aside.

3. Add clams to the pan, cover, cook over medium-high heat until they open, transfer to the bowl with mussels, and leave aside. Add squid to the pan, cover and cook over medium-high heat for 3 minutes, transfer to the bowl with mussels and clams.

4. Meanwhile, slice octopus into small pieces and mix with the rest of the seafood. Add sliced celery, radicchio, red onion, vinegar, olive oil, parsley, salt, and pepper, stir gently, and leave aside in the fridge within 2 hours before serving.

Nutrition:

Calories: 102; Carbs: 7g; Fat: 1g; Protein: 16g; Sodium: 0mg

Shrimp and Onion Ginger Dressing

Preparation time: 10 minutes

Cooking time: 5 minutes

Servings: 2

Ingredients:

- 8 medium shrimp, peeled and deveined
- 12 ounces package mixed salad leaves
- 10 cherry tomatoes, halved
- 2 green onions, sliced
- 2 medium mushrooms, sliced
- 1/3 cup rice vinegar
- ¼ cup sesame seeds, toasted
- 1 tablespoon low-sodium soy sauce
- 2 teaspoons ginger, grated
- 2 teaspoons garlic, minced
- 2/3 cup canola oil
- 1/3 cup sesame oil

Directions:

1. In a bowl, mix rice vinegar with sesame seeds, soy sauce, garlic, ginger, and stir well. Pour this into your kitchen blender, add canola oil and sesame oil, pulse very well, and leave aside. Brush shrimp with 3 tablespoons of the ginger dressing you've prepared.
2. Heat your kitchen grill over high heat, add shrimp and cook for 3 minutes, flipping once. In a salad bowl, mix salad leaves with grilled shrimp, mushrooms, green onions, and tomatoes. Drizzle ginger dressing on top and serve right away!

Nutrition:

Calories: 360; Carbs: 14g; Fat: 11g; Protein: 49g; Sodium: 469 mg

Fruit Shrimp Soup

Preparation time: 10 minutes
Cooking time: 25 minutes
Servings: 6
Ingredients:

- 8 ounces shrimp, peeled and deveined
- 1 stalk lemongrass, smashed
- 2 small ginger pieces, grated
- 6 cup chicken stock
- 2 jalapenos, chopped
- 4 lime leaves
- 1 and ½ cups pineapple, chopped
- 1 cup shiitake mushroom caps, chopped
- 1 tomato, chopped
- ½ bell pepper, cubed
- 2 tablespoons fish sauce
- 1 teaspoon sugar
- ¼ cup lime juice
- 1/3 cup cilantro, chopped
- 2 scallions, sliced

Directions:

1. In a pot, mix ginger with lemongrass, stock, jalapenos, and lime leaves, stir, boil over medium heat, cook within 15 minutes. Strain liquid in a bowl and discard solids.
2. Return soup to the pot again, add pineapple, tomato, mushrooms, bell pepper, sugar, and fish sauce, stir, boil over medium heat, cook for 5 minutes, add shrimp and cook for 3 more minutes. Remove from heat, add lime juice, cilantro, and scallions, stir, ladle into soup bowls and serve.

Nutrition:
Calories: 290; Carbs: 39g; Fat: 12g; Protein: 7g; Sodium: 21 mg

Mussels and Chickpea Soup

Preparation time: 10 minutes
Cooking time: 10 minutes
Servings: 6
Ingredients:

- 3 garlic cloves, minced
- 2 tablespoons olive oil
- A pinch of chili flakes
- 1 and ½ tablespoons fresh mussels, scrubbed
- 1 cup white wine
- 1 cup chickpeas, rinsed
- 1 small fennel bulb, sliced
- Black pepper to the taste
- Juice of 1 lemon
- 3 tablespoons parsley, chopped

Directions:

1. Heat a big saucepan with the olive oil over medium-high heat, add garlic and chili flakes, stir and cook within a couple of minutes. Add white wine and mussels, stir, cover, and cook for 3-4 minutes until mussels open.
2. Transfer mussels to a baking dish, add some of the cooking liquid over them, and fridge until they are cold enough. Take mussels out of the fridge and discard shells.
3. Heat another pan over medium-high heat, add mussels, reserved cooking liquid, chickpeas, and fennel, stir well, and heat them. Add black pepper to the taste, lemon juice, and parsley, stir again, divide between plates and serve.

Nutrition:
Calories: 286; Carbs: 49g; Fat: 4g; Protein: 14g; Sodium: 145mg

Fish Stew

Preparation time: 10 minutes
Cooking time: 30 minutes
Servings: 4
Ingredients:

- 1 red onion, sliced
- 2 tablespoons olive oil
- 1-pound white fish fillets, boneless, skinless, and cubed
- 1 avocado, pitted and chopped
- 1 tablespoon oregano, chopped
- 1 cup chicken stock
- 2 tomatoes, cubed
- 1 teaspoon sweet paprika
- A pinch of salt and black pepper
- 1 tablespoon parsley, chopped
- Juice of 1 lime

Directions:

1. Warm-up oil in a pot over medium heat, add the onion, and sauté within 5 minutes. Add the fish, the avocado, and the other ingredients, toss, cook over medium heat for 25 minutes more, divide into bowls and serve for lunch.

Nutrition:
Calories: 78; Carbs: 8g; Fat: 1g; Protein: 11g; Sodium: 151 mg

Shrimp and Broccoli Soup

Preparation time: 5 minutes
Cooking time: 25 minutes
Servings: 4
Ingredients:
- 2 tablespoons olive oil
- 1 yellow onion, chopped
- 4 cups chicken stock
- Juice of 1 lime
- 1-pound shrimp, peeled and deveined
- ½ cup coconut cream
- ½ pound broccoli florets
- 1 tablespoon parsley, chopped

Directions:
1. Heat a pot with the oil over medium heat, add the onion and sauté for 5 minutes. Add the shrimp and the other ingredients, simmer over medium heat for 20 minutes more. Ladle the soup into bowls and serve.

Nutrition:
Calories: 220; Carbs: 12g; Fat: 7g; Protein: 26g; Sodium: 577 mg

Coconut Turkey Mix

Preparation time: 10 minutes
Cooking time: 30 minutes
Servings: 4
Ingredients:

- 1 yellow onion, chopped
- 1-pound turkey breast, skinless, boneless, and cubed
- 2 tablespoons olive oil
- 2 garlic cloves, minced
- 1 zucchini, sliced
- 1 cup coconut cream
- A pinch of sea salt
- black pepper

Directions:

1. Bring the pan to medium heat, add the onion and the garlic and sauté for 5 minutes. Put the meat and brown within 5 minutes more. Add the rest of the ingredients, toss, bring to a simmer and cook over medium heat for 20 minutes more. Serve for lunch.

Nutrition:

Calories 200; Fat 4g; Fiber 2g; Carbs 14g; Protein 7g; Sodium 111mg

Lime Shrimp and Kale

Preparation time: 10 minutes
Cooking time: 20 minutes
Servings: 4
Ingredients:
- 1-pound shrimp, peeled and deveined
- 4 scallions, chopped
- 1 teaspoon sweet paprika
- 1 tablespoon olive oil
- Juice of 1 lime
- Zest of 1 lime, grated
- A pinch of salt and black pepper
- 2 tablespoons parsley, chopped

Directions:
1. Bring the pan to medium heat, add the scallions and sauté for 5 minutes. Add the shrimp and the other ingredients, toss, cook over medium heat for 15 minutes more, divide into bowls and serve.

Nutrition:
Calories: 149; Carbs: 12g; Fat: 4g; Protein: 21g; Sodium: 250 mg

Parsley Cod Mix

Preparation time: 10 minutes
Cooking time: 20 minutes
Servings: 4
Ingredients:

- 1 tablespoon olive oil
- 2 shallots, chopped
- 4 cod fillets, boneless and skinless
- 2 garlic cloves, minced
- 2 tablespoons lemon juice
- 1 cup chicken stock
- A pinch of salt and black pepper

Directions:

1. Bring the pan to medium heat -high heat, add the shallots and the garlic and sauté for 5 minutes. Add the cod and the other ingredients, cook everything for 15 minutes more, divide between plates and serve for lunch.

Nutrition:
Calories: 216; Carbs: 7g; Fat: 5g; Protein: 34g; Sodium: 380 mg

Salmon and Cabbage Mix

Preparation time: 5 minutes

Cooking time: 25 minutes

Servings: 4

Ingredients:

- 4 salmon fillets, boneless
- 1 yellow onion, chopped
- 2 tablespoons olive oil
- 1 cup red cabbage, shredded
- 1 red bell pepper, chopped
- 1 tablespoon rosemary, chopped
- 1 tablespoon coriander, ground
- 1 cup tomato sauce
- A pinch of sea salt
- black pepper

Directions:

1. Bring the pan to medium heat, add the onion and sauté for 5 minutes. Put the fish and sear it within 2 minutes on each side. Add the cabbage and the remaining ingredients, toss, cook over medium heat for 20 minutes more, divide between plates and serve.

Nutrition:

Calories: 130; Carbs: 8g; Fat: 6g; Protein: 12g; Sodium: 345 mg

Decent Beef and Onion Stew

Preparation time: 10 minutes
Cooking time: 1-2 hours
Servings: 4
Ingredients:
- 2 pounds lean beef, cubed
- 3 pounds shallots, peeled
- 5 garlic cloves, peeled, whole
- 3 tablespoons tomato paste
- 1 bay leaves
- ¼ cup olive oil
- 3 tablespoons lemon juice

Directions:
1. Take a stew pot and place it over medium heat.
2. Add olive oil and let it heat up.
3. Add meat and brown.
4. Add remaining ingredients and cover with water.
5. Bring the whole mix to a boil.
6. Reduce heat to low and cover the pot.
7. Simmer for 1-2 hours until beef is cooked thoroughly.
8. Serve hot!

Nutrition:
Calories: 136; Fat: 3g; Carbohydrates: 0.9g; Protein: 24g

Clean Parsley and Chicken Breast

Preparation time: 10 minutes
Cooking time: 40 minutes
Servings: 2
Ingredients:

- 1/2 tablespoon dry parsley
- 1/2 tablespoon dry basil
- 2 chicken breast halves, boneless and skinless
- 1/4 teaspoon sunflower seeds
- 1/4 teaspoon red pepper flakes, crushed
- 1 tomato, sliced

Directions:

1. Pre-heat your oven to 350 degrees F.
2. Take a 9x13 inch baking dish and grease it up with cooking spray.
3. Sprinkle 1 tablespoon of parsley, 1 teaspoon of basil and spread the mixture over your baking dish.
4. Arrange the chicken breast halves over the dish and sprinkle garlic slices on top.
5. Take a small bowl and add 1 teaspoon parsley, 1 teaspoon of basil, sunflower seeds, basil, and red pepper and mix well. Pour the mixture over the chicken breast.
6. Top with tomato slices and cover, bake for 25 minutes.
7. Remove the cover and bake for 15 minutes more.
8. Serve and enjoy!

Nutrition:
Calories: 150; Fat: 4g; Carbohydrates: 4g; Protein: 25g

Zucchini Beef Sauté with Coriander Greens

Preparation time: 10 minutes

Cooking time: 10 minutes

Servings: 4

Ingredients:

- 10 ounces beef, sliced into 1–2-inch strips
- 1 zucchini, cut into 2-inch strips
- ¼ cup parsley, chopped
- 3 garlic cloves, minced
- 2 tablespoons tamari sauce
- 4 tablespoons avocado oil

Directions:

1. Add 2 tablespoons avocado oil in a frying pan over high heat.
2. Place strips of beef and brown for a few minutes on high heat.
3. Once the meat is brown, add zucchini strips and sauté until tender.
4. Once tender, add tamari sauce, garlic, parsley and let them sit for a few minutes more.
5. Serve immediately and enjoy!

Nutrition:

Calories: 500; Fat: 40g; Carbohydrates: 5g; Protein: 31g

Hearty Lemon and Pepper Chicken

Preparation time: 5 minutes
Cooking time: 15 minutes
Servings: 4
Ingredients:

- 2 teaspoons olive oil
- 1 ¼ pounds skinless chicken cutlets
- 2 whole eggs
- ¼ cup panko crumbs
- 1 tablespoon lemon pepper
- Sunflower seeds and pepper to taste
- 3 cups green beans
- ¼ cup parmesan cheese
- ¼ teaspoon garlic powder

Directions:

1. Pre-heat your oven to 425 degrees F.
2. Take a bowl and stir in seasoning, parmesan, lemon pepper, garlic powder, panko.
3. Whisk eggs in another bowl.
4. Coat cutlets in eggs and press into panko mix.
5. Transfer coated chicken to a parchment lined baking sheet.
6. Toss the beans in oil, pepper, add sunflower seeds, and lay them on the side of the baking sheet.
7. Bake for 15 minutes.
8. Enjoy!

Nutrition:
Calorie: 299; Fat: 10g; Carbohydrates: 10g; Protein: 43g

Walnuts and Asparagus Delight

Preparation time: 5 minutes

Cooking time: 5 minutes

Servings: 4

Ingredients:

- 1 ½ tablespoons olive oil
- ¾ pound asparagus, trimmed
- ¼ cup walnuts, chopped
- Sunflower seeds and pepper to taste

Directions:

1. Place a skillet over medium heat add olive oil and let it heat up.
2. Add asparagus, sauté for 5 minutes until browned. Season with sunflower seeds and pepper. Remove heat. Add walnuts and toss. Serve warm!

Nutrition:

Calories: 124; Fat: 12g; Carbohydrates: 2g; Protein: 3g

Healthy Carrot Chips

Preparation time: 10 minutes

Cooking time: 10 minutes

Servings: 4

Ingredients:

- 3 cups carrots, sliced paper-thin rounds
- 2 tablespoons olive oil
- 2 teaspoons ground cumin
- ½ teaspoon smoked paprika
- Pinch of sunflower seeds

Directions:

1. Pre-heat your oven to 400 degrees F.
2. Slice carrot into paper thin shaped coins using a peeler.
3. Place slices in a bowl and toss with oil and spices.
4. Lay out the slices on a parchment paper, lined baking sheet in a single layer.
5. Sprinkle sunflower seeds.
6. Transfer to oven and bake for 8-10 minutes.
7. Remove and serve.
8. Enjoy!

Nutrition:

Calories: 434; Fat: 35g; Carbohydrates: 31g; Protein: 2g

Beef Soup

Preparation time: 10 minutes
Cooking time: 40 minutes
Servings: 4
Ingredients:
- 1 pound ground beef, lean
- 1 cup mixed vegetables, frozen
- 1 yellow onion, chopped
- 6 cups vegetable broth
- 1 cup low-fat cream
- Pepper to taste

Directions:
1. Take a stockpot and add all the ingredients the except heavy cream, salt, and black pepper.
2. Bring to a boil.
3. Reduce heat to simmer.
4. Cook for 40 minutes.
5. Once cooked, warm the heavy cream.
6. Then add once the soup is cooked.
7. Blend the soup till smooth by using an immersion blender.
8. Season with salt and black pepper.
9. Serve and enjoy!

Nutrition:
Calories: 270; Fat: 14g; Carbohydrates: 6g; Protein: 29g

CHAPTER 7:

Sides

Tomatoes Side Salad

Preparation time: 10 minutes
Cooking time: 0 minutes
Servings: 4

Ingredients:

- ½ bunch mint, chopped
- 8 plum tomatoes, sliced
- 1 teaspoon mustard
- 1 tablespoon rosemary vinegar
- A pinch of black pepper

Directions:

1. In a bowl, mix vinegar with mustard and pepper and whisk.
2. In another bowl, combine the tomatoes with the mint and the vinaigrette, toss, divide between plates and serve as a side dish.
3. Enjoy!

Nutrition: calories 70, fat 2, fiber 2, carbs 6, protein 4

Squash Salsa

Preparation time: 10 minutes
Cooking time: 13 minutes
Servings: 6

Ingredients:

- 3 tablespoons olive oil
- 5 medium squash, peeled and sliced
- 1 cup pepitas, toasted
- 7 tomatillos
- A pinch of black pepper
- 1 small onion, chopped
- 2 tablespoons fresh lime juice
- 2 tablespoons cilantro, chopped

Directions:

1. Heat up a pan over medium heat, add tomatillos, onion and black pepper, stir, cook for 3 minutes, transfer to your food processor and pulse.
2. Add lime juice and cilantro, pulse again and transfer to a bowl.
3. Heat up your kitchen grill over high heat, drizzle the oil over squash slices, grill them for 10 minutes, divide them between plates, add pepitas and tomatillos mix on top and serve as a side dish.
4. Enjoy!

Nutrition: calories 120, fat 2, fiber 1, carbs 7, protein 1

Apples and Fennel Mix

Preparation time: 10 minutes
Cooking time: 0 minutes
Servings: 3
Ingredients:
- 3 big apples, cored and sliced
- 1 and ½ cup fennel, shredded
- 1/3 cup coconut cream
- 3 tablespoons apple vinegar
- ½ teaspoon caraway seeds
- Black pepper to the taste

Directions:
1. In a bowl, mix fennel with apples and toss.
2. In another bowl, mix coconut cream with vinegar, black pepper and caraway seeds, whisk well, add over the fennel mix, toss, divide between plates and serve as a side dish. Enjoy!

Nutrition: calories 130, fat 3, fiber 6, carbs 10, protein 3

Simple Roasted Celery Mix

Preparation time: 10 minutes
Cooking time: 25 minutes
Servings: 3

Ingredients:

- 3 celery roots, cubed
- 2 tablespoons olive oil
- A pinch of black pepper
- 2 cups natural and unsweetened apple juice - ¼ cup parsley, chopped
- ¼ cup walnuts, chopped

Directions:

1. In a baking dish, combine the celery with the oil, pepper, parsley, walnuts and apple juice, toss to coat, introduce in the oven at 450 degrees F, bake for 25 minutes, divide between plates and serve as a side dish. Enjoy!

Nutrition: calories 140, fat 2, fiber 2, carbs 7, protein 7

Thyme Spring Onions

Preparation time: 10 minutes

Cooking time: 40 minutes

Servings: 8

Ingredients:

- 15 spring onions
- A pinch of black pepper
- 1 teaspoon thyme, chopped
- 1 tablespoon olive oil

Directions:

1. Put onions in a baking dish, add thyme, black pepper and oil, toss, bake in the oven at 350 degrees F for 40 minutes, divide between plates and serve as a side dish. Enjoy!

Nutrition: calories 120, fat 2, fiber 2, carbs 7, protein 2

Carrot Slaw

Preparation time: 10 minutes
Cooking time: 10 minutes
Servings: 4
Ingredients:
- ¼ yellow onion, chopped
- 5 carrots, cut into thin matchsticks
- 1 tablespoon olive oil
- 1 garlic clove, minced
- 1 tablespoon Dijon mustard
- 1 tablespoon red vinegar
- A pinch of black pepper
- 1 tablespoon lemon juice

Directions:
1. In a bowl, mix vinegar with black pepper, mustard and lemon juice and whisk.
2. Heat up a pan with the oil over medium heat, add onion, stir and cook for 5 minutes.
3. Add garlic and carrots, stir, cook for 5 minutes more, transfer to a salad bowl, cool down, add the vinaigrette, toss, divide between plates and serve as a side dish. Enjoy!

Nutrition: calories 120, fat 3, fiber 3, carbs 7, protein 5

Watermelon Tomato Salsa

Preparation time: 10 minutes
Cooking time: 0 minutes
Servings: 16

Ingredients:

- 4 yellow tomatoes, seedless and chopped
- A pinch of black pepper
- 1 cup watermelon, seedless and chopped
- 1/3 cup red onion, chopped
- 2 jalapeno peppers, chopped
- ¼ cup cilantro, chopped
- 3 tablespoons lime juice

Directions:

1. In a bowl, mix tomatoes with watermelon, onion and jalapeno.
2. Add cilantro, lime juice and pepper, toss, divide between plates and serve as a side dish.
3. Enjoy!

Nutrition: calories 87, fat 1, fiber 2, carbs 4, protein 7

Sprouts Side Salad

Preparation time: 10 minutes

Cooking time: 0 minutes

Servings: 4

Ingredients:

- 2 zucchinis, cut with a spiralizer
- 2 cups bean sprouts
- 4 green onions, chopped
- 1 red bell pepper, chopped
- Juice of 1 lime
- 1 tablespoon olive oil
- ½ cup cilantro, chopped
- ¾ cup almonds, chopped
- Black pepper to the taste

Directions:

1. In a salad bowl, mix zucchinis with bean sprouts, onions and bell pepper.
2. Add black pepper, lime juice, almonds, cilantro and olive oil, toss everything, divide between plates and serve as a side dish.
3. Enjoy!

Nutrition: calories 120, fat 4, fiber 2, carbs 7, protein 12

Cabbage Slaw

Preparation time: 10 minutes

Cooking time: 0 minutes

Servings: 4

Ingredients:

- 1 green cabbage head, shredded
- 1/3 cup coconut, shredded
- ¼ cup olive oil
- 2 tablespoons lemon juice
- ¼ cup coconut aminos
- 3 tablespoons sesame seeds
- ½ teaspoon curry powder
- 1/3 teaspoon turmeric powder
- ½ teaspoon cumin, ground

Directions:

1. In a bowl, mix cabbage with coconut and lemon juice and stir.
2. Add oil, aminos, sesame seeds, curry powder, turmeric and cumin, toss to coat and serve as a side dish.
3. Enjoy!

Nutrition: calories 130, fat 4, fiber 5, carbs 8, protein 6

Edamame Side Salad

Preparation time: 10 minutes
Cooking time: 0 minutes
Servings: 4
Ingredients:
- 1 tablespoon ginger, grated
- 2 green onions, chopped
- 3 cups edamame, blanched
- 2 tablespoons rice vinegar
- 1 tablespoon sesame seeds

Directions:
1. In a bowl, combine the ginger with the onions, edamame, vinegar and sesame seeds, toss, divide between plates and serve as a side dish.
2. Enjoy!

Nutrition: calories 120, fat 3, fiber 2, carbs 5, protein 9

Flavored Beets Side Salad

Preparation time: 10 minutes
Cooking time: 0 minutes
Servings: 4

Ingredients:

- 4 carrots, sliced
- 12 radishes, sliced
- 1 beet, peeled and grated
- 2 tablespoons raisins
- Juice of 2 lemons
- 1 sugar beet, peeled and chopped
- 1 tablespoon chives, chopped
- 1 tablespoon parsley, chopped
- 1 tablespoon lemon thyme, chopped
- 1 tablespoon white sesame seeds
- 4 handfuls spinach leaves
- 4 tablespoons olive oil
- Black pepper to the taste

Directions:

1. In a salad bowl, mix carrots, radishes, beets, sugar beet, raisins, chives, parsley, spinach, thyme and sesame seeds.
2. Add lemon juice, oil and black pepper, toss well and serve as a side dish.
3. Enjoy!

Nutrition: calories 110, fat 2, fiber 2, carbs 4, protein 7

Tomato and Avocado Salad

Preparation time: 10 minutes
Cooking time: 0 minutes
Servings: 4
Ingredients:

- 1 cucumber, chopped
- 1-pound tomatoes, chopped
- 2 avocados, pitted, peeled and chopped
- 1 small red onion, sliced
- 2 tablespoons olive oil
- 2 tablespoons lemon juice
- ¼ cup cilantro, chopped
- Black pepper to the taste

Directions:

1. In a salad bowl, mix tomatoes with onion, avocado, cucumber and cilantro.
2. In a small bowl, mix oil with lemon juice and black pepper, whisk well, pour this over the salad, toss and serve as a side dish.
3. Enjoy!

Nutrition: calories 120, fat 2, fiber 2, carbs 3, protein 4

Greek Side Salad

Preparation time: 10 minutes
Cooking time: 0 minutes
Servings: 4

Ingredients:

- 4 pounds heirloom tomatoes, sliced
- 1 yellow bell pepper, thinly sliced
- 1 green bell pepper, thinly sliced
- 1 red onion, thinly sliced
- Black pepper to the taste
- ½ teaspoon oregano, dried
- 2 tablespoons mint leaves, chopped
- A drizzle of olive oil

Directions:

1. In a salad bowl, mix tomatoes with yellow and green peppers, onion, salt and pepper, toss to coat and leave aside for 10 minutes.
2. Add oregano, mint and olive oil, toss to coat and serve as a side salad.
3. Enjoy!

Nutrition: calories 100, fat 2, fiber 2, carbs 3, protein 6

Cucumber Salad

Preparation time: 10 minutes

Cooking time: 0 minutes

Servings: 4

Ingredients:

- 2 English cucumbers, chopped
- 8 dates, pitted and sliced
- ¾ cup fennel, sliced
- 2 tablespoons chives, chopped
- ½ cup walnuts, chopped
- 2 tablespoons lemon juice
- 4 tablespoons olive oil
- Black pepper to the taste

Directions:

1. In a salad bowl, combine the cucumbers with dates, fennel, chives, walnuts, lemon juice, oil and black pepper, toss, divide between plates and serve as a side dish.
2. Enjoy!

Nutrition: calories 100, fat 1, fiber 1, carbs 7, protein 6

Black Beans and Veggies Side Salad

Preparation time: 10 minutes
Cooking time: 0 minutes
Servings: 4
Ingredients:

- 1 big cucumber, cut into chunks
- 15 ounces canned black beans, no-salt-added, drained and rinsed
- 1 cup corn
- 1 cup cherry tomatoes, halved
- 1 small red onion, chopped
- 3 tablespoons olive oil
- 4 and ½ teaspoons orange marmalade
- Black pepper to the taste
- ½ teaspoon cumin, ground
- 1 tablespoon lemon juice

Directions:

1. In a bowl, mix beans with cucumber, corn, onion and tomatoes.
2. In another bowl, mix marmalade with oil, lemon juice, black pepper to the taste and cumin, whisk, pour over the salad, toss and serve as a side dish.
3. Enjoy!

Nutrition: calories 110, fat 0, fiber 3, carbs 6, protein 8

Endives and Escarole Side Salad

Preparation time: 10 minutes

Cooking time: 0 minutes

Servings: 4

Ingredients:

- 1 teaspoon shallot, minced
- ¼ cup apple cider vinegar
- 1 teaspoon Dijon mustard
- 3 Belgian endives, roughly chopped
- ¾ cup olive oil
- 1 cup escarole leaves, torn

Directions:

1. In a bowl, mix escarole leaves with endives, shallot, vinegar, mustard and oil, toss, divide between plates and serve as a side salad. Enjoy!

Nutrition: calories 100, fat 1, fiber 3, carbs 6, protein 7

Radicchio and Lettuce Side Salad

Preparation time: 10 minutes

Cooking time: 0 minutes

Servings: 4

Ingredients:

- ½ cup olive oil
- Black pepper to the taste
- 2 tablespoons shallot, chopped
- ¼ cup mustard
- Juice of 2 lemons
- ½ cup basil, chopped
- 5 baby romaine lettuce heads, chopped
- 3 radicchios, sliced
- 3 endives, roughly chopped

Directions:

1. In a salad bowl, mix romaine lettuce with radicchios and endives.
2. In another bowl, mix oil with the pepper, shallot, mustard, lemon juice and basil, whisk, add to the salad, toss and serve as a side salad. Enjoy!

Nutrition: calories 120, fat 2, fiber 1, carbs 8, protein 2

Jicama Side Salad

Preparation time: 10 minutes
Cooking time: 0 minutes
Servings: 4
Ingredients:

- 1 romaine lettuce head, leaves torn
- 1 Jicama, peeled and grated
- 1 cup cherry tomatoes, halved
- 1 yellow bell pepper, chopped
- 1 cup carrot, shredded
- 3 ounces low-fat cheese, crumbled
- 3 tablespoons red wine vinegar
- 5 tablespoons non-fat yogurt
- 1 and ½ tablespoons olive oil
- 1 teaspoon parsley, chopped
- 1 teaspoon dill, chopped
- Black pepper to the taste

Directions:

1. In a salad bowl, mix lettuce leaves with Jicama, tomatoes, bell pepper and carrot and toss.
2. In another bowl, combine the cheese with vinegar, yogurt, oil, pepper, dill and parsley, whisk, add to the salad, toss to coat, divide between plates and serve as a side dish.
3. Enjoy!

Nutrition: calories 170, fat 4, fiber 8, carbs 14, protein 11

Cauliflower Risotto

Preparation time: 10 minutes
Cooking time: 7 minutes
Servings: 4
Ingredients:

- 2 tablespoons olive oil
- 2 garlic cloves, minced
- 12 ounces cauliflower rice
- 2 tablespoons thyme, chopped
- 1 tablespoon lemon juice
- Zest of ½ lemon, grated
- A pinch of black pepper

Directions:

1. Heat up a pan with the oil over medium-high heat, add cauliflower rice and garlic, stir and cook for 5 minutes.
2. Add lemon juice, lemon zest, thyme, salt and pepper, stir, cook for 2 minutes more, divide between plates and serve as a side dish.
3. Enjoy!

Nutrition: calories 130, fat 2, fiber 2, carbs 6, protein 8

Three Beans Mix

Preparation time: 10 minutes
Cooking time: 0 minutes
Servings: 4
Ingredients:

- 15 ounces canned kidney beans, no-salt-added, drained and rinsed
- 15 ounces canned garbanzo beans, no-salt-added and drained
- 15 ounces canned pinto beans, no-salt- added and drained
- 3 tablespoons balsamic vinegar
- 2 tablespoons olive oil
- 2 teaspoon Italian seasoning
- 2 teaspoons garlic powder
- 1 teaspoon onion powder

Directions:

1. In a large salad bowl, combine the beans with vinegar, oil, seasoning, garlic powder and onion powder, toss, divide between plates and serve as a side dish. Enjoy!

Nutrition: calories 140, fat 1, fiber 10, carbs 10, protein 7

Cranberry and Broccoli Mix

Preparation time: 10 minutes
Cooking time: 0 minutes
Servings: 4
Ingredients:

- ½ cup avocado mayonnaise
- 1 tablespoon apple cider vinegar
- 1 tablespoon lemon juice
- 1 tablespoon coconut sugar
- ¼ cup cranberries
- ½ cup almonds, sliced
- 9 ounces broccoli florets, separated

Directions:

1. In a bowl, mix broccoli with cranberries and almond slices and toss.
2. In another bowl, mix coconut sugar with vinegar, mayo and lemon juice, whisk well, add to the broccoli mix, toss, divide between plates and serve as a side dish.
3. Enjoy!

Nutrition: calories 120, fat 1, fiber 3, carbs 7, protein 8

Bell Peppers Mix

Preparation time: 10 minutes

Cooking time: 10 minutes

Servings: 2

Ingredients:

- 1 tablespoon olive oil
- 2 teaspoons garlic powder
- 2 red bell peppers, chopped
- 2 yellow bell peppers, chopped
- 2 orange bell peppers, chopped
- Black pepper to the taste

Directions:

1. Heat up a pan with the oil over medium-high heat, add all the bell peppers, stir and cook for 5 minutes.
2. Add garlic powder and black pepper, stir, cook for 5 minutes, divide between plates and serve as a side dish.
3. Enjoy!

Nutrition: calories 145, fat 3, fiber 5, carbs 5, protein 8

Sweet Potato Mash

Preparation time: 10 minutes
Cooking time: 1 hour
Servings: 6

Ingredients:
- ¼ cup olive oil
- 3 pounds sweet potatoes
- Black pepper to the taste

Directions:
1. Arrange the sweet potatoes on a lined baking sheet, introduce in the oven, bake at 375 degrees F for 1 hour, cool them down, peel, mash them and put them in a bowl.
2. Add black pepper and the oil, whisk well, divide between plates and serve as a side dish.
3. Enjoy!

Nutrition: calories 140, fat 1, fiber 4, carbs 6, protein 4

Creamy Cucumber Mix

Preparation time: 10 minutes
Cooking time: 0 minutes
Servings: 2

Ingredients:

- 1 big cucumber, peeled and chopped
- 1 small red onion, chopped
- 4 tablespoons non-fat yogurt
- 1 teaspoon balsamic vinegar

Directions:

1. In a bowl, mix onion with cucumber, yogurt and vinegar, toss, divide between plates and serve as a side dish.
2. Enjoy!

Nutrition: calories 90, fat 1, fiber 3, carbs 7, protein 2

Bok Choy Mix

Preparation time: 10 minutes
Cooking time: 15 minutes
Servings: 4
Ingredients:

- 2 tablespoons olive oil
- 3 tablespoons coconut aminos
- 1-inch ginger, grated
- A pinch of red pepper flakes
- 4 bok choy heads, cut into quarters
- 2 garlic cloves, minced
- 1 tablespoon sesame seeds, toasted

Directions:

1. Heat up a pan with the olive oil over medium heat, add coconut aminos, garlic, pepper flakes and ginger, stir and cook for 3-4 minutes.
2. Add the bok choy and the sesame seeds, toss, cook for 5 minutes more, divide between plates and serve as a side dish.
3. Enjoy!

Nutrition: calories 140, fat 2, fiber 2, carbs 4, protein 6

Flavored Turnips Mix

Preparation time: 10 minutes
Cooking time: 15 minutes
Servings: 4

Ingredients:
- 1 tablespoon lemon juice
- Zest of 2 oranges, grated
- 16 ounces turnips, sliced
- 3 tablespoons olive oil
- 1 tablespoon rosemary, chopped
- Black pepper to the taste

Directions:
1. Heat up a pan with the oil over medium-high heat, add turnips, stir and cook for 5 minutes.
2. Add lemon juice, black pepper, orange zest and rosemary, stir, cook for 10 minutes more, divide between plates and serve as a side dish.
3. Enjoy!

Nutrition: calories 130, fat 1, fiber 2, carbs 8, protein 4

Lemony Fennel Mix

Preparation time: 10 minutes
Cooking time: 0 minutes
Servings: 4

Ingredients:

- 3 tablespoons lemon juice
- 1 pound fennel, chopped
- 2 tablespoons olive oil
- A pinch of black pepper

Directions:

1. In a salad bowl, mix fennel with and black pepper, oil and lemon juice, toss well, divide between plates and serve as a side dish.
2. Enjoy!

Nutrition: calories 130, fat 1, fiber 1, carbs 7, protein 7

Simple Cauliflower Mix

Preparation time: 10 minutes
Cooking time: 35 minutes
Servings: 4
Ingredients:

- 6 cups cauliflower florets
- 2 teaspoons sweet paprika
- 2 cups chicken stock
- ¼ cup avocado oil
- Black pepper to the taste

Directions:

1. In a baking dish, combine the cauliflower with stock, oil, black pepper and paprika, toss, introduce in the oven and bake at 375 degrees F for 35 minutes.
2. Divide between plates and serve as a side dish.
3. Enjoy!

Nutrition: calories 180, fat 3, fiber 2, carbs 46, protein 6

Broccoli Mix

Preparation time: 10 minutes
Cooking time: 3 hours
Servings: 10
Ingredients:
- 6 cups broccoli florets
- 10 ounces tomato sauce, sodium-free
- 1 and ½ cups low-fat cheddar cheese, shredded
- ½ teaspoon cider vinegar
- ¼ cup yellow onion, chopped
- A pinch of black pepper
- 2 tablespoons olive oil

Directions:
1. Grease your slow cooker with the oil, add broccoli, tomato sauce, cider vinegar, onion and black pepper, cover and cook on High for 2 hours and 30 minutes.
2. Sprinkle the cheese all over, cover, cook on High for 30 minutes more, divide between plates and serve as a side dish.
3. Enjoy!

Nutrition: calories 160, fat 6, fiber 4, carbs 11, protein 6

Tasty Bean Side Dish

Preparation time: 10 minutes

Cooking time: 5 hours

Servings: 10

Ingredients:

- 1 and ½ cups tomato sauce, salt-free
- 1 yellow onion, chopped
- 2 celery ribs, chopped
- 1 sweet red pepper, chopped
- 1 green bell pepper, chopped
- ½ cup water
- 2 bay leaves

- 1 teaspoon ground mustard
- 1 tablespoon cider vinegar
- 16 ounces canned kidney beans, no-salt-added, drained and rinsed
- 16 ounces canned black-eyed peas, no-salt-added, drained and rinsed
- 15 ounces corn
- 15 ounces canned lima beans, no-salt-added, drained and rinsed
- 15 ounces canned black beans, no-salt-added, drained and rinsed

Directions:

1. In your slow cooker, mix the tomato sauce with the onion, celery, red pepper, green bell pepper, water, bay leaves, mustard, vinegar, kidney beans, black-eyed peas, corn, lima beans and black beans, cover and cook on Low for 5 hours.
2. Discard bay leaves, divide the whole mix between plates and serve.
3. Enjoy!

Nutrition: calories 211, fat 4, fiber 8, carbs 20, protein 7

Easy Green Beans

Preparation time: 10 minutes

Cooking time: 2 hours

Servings: 12

Ingredients:

- 16 ounces green beans
- 3 tablespoons olive oil
- ½ cup coconut sugar
- 1 teaspoon low-sodium soy sauce
- ½ teaspoon garlic powder

Directions:

1. In your slow cooker, mix the green beans with the oil, sugar, soy sauce and garlic powder, cover and cook on Low for 2 hours.
2. Toss the beans, divide them between plates and serve as a side dish.
3. Enjoy!

Nutrition: calories 142, fat 7, fiber 4, carbs 15, protein 3

Creamy Corn

Preparation time: 10 minutes
Cooking time: 4 hours
Servings: 12

Ingredients:

- 10 cups corn
- 20 ounces fat-free cream cheese
- ½ cup fat-free milk
- ½ cup low-fat butter
- A pinch of black pepper
- 2 tablespoons green onions, chopped

Directions:

1. In your slow cooker, mix the corn with cream cheese, milk, butter, black pepper and onions, toss, cover and cook on Low for 4 hours.
2. Toss one more time, divide between plates and serve as a side dish.
3. Enjoy!

Nutrition: calories 256, fat 11, fiber 2, carbs 17, protein 5

Classic Peas and Carrots

Preparation time: 10 minutes

Cooking time: 5 hours

Servings: 12

Ingredients:

- 1-pound carrots, sliced
- ¼ cup water
- 1 yellow onion, chopped
- 2 tablespoons olive oil
- 2 tablespoons stevia
- 4 garlic cloves, minced
- 1 teaspoon marjoram, dried
- A pinch of white pepper
- 16 ounces peas

Directions:

1. In your slow cooker, mix the carrots with water, onion, oil, stevia, garlic, marjoram, white pepper and peas, toss, cover and cook on High for 5 hours.
2. Divide between plates and serve as a side dish.
3. Enjoy!

Nutrition: calories 107, fat 3, fiber 3, carbs 14, protein 4

Mushroom Pilaf

Preparation time: 10 minutes
Cooking time: 3 hours
Servings: 6
Ingredients:
- 1 cup wild rice
- 2 garlic cloves, minced
- 6 green onions, chopped
- 2 tablespoons olive oil
- ½ pound baby Bella mushrooms
- 2 cups water

Directions:
1. In your slow cooker, mix the rice with garlic, onions, oil, mushrooms and water, toss, cover and cook on Low for 3 hours.
2. Stir the pilaf one more time, divide between plates and serve. Enjoy!

Nutrition: calories 210, fat 7, fiber 1, carbs 16, protein 4

Butternut Mix

Preparation time: 10 minutes
Cooking time: 4 hours
Servings: 8

Ingredients:

- 1 cup carrots, chopped
- 1 tablespoon olive oil
- 1 yellow onion, chopped
- ½ teaspoon stevia
- 1 garlic clove, minced
- ½ teaspoon curry powder
- ½ teaspoon cinnamon powder
- ¼ teaspoon ginger, grated
- 1 butternut squash, cubed
- 2 and ½ cups low-sodium veggie stock
- ½ cup basmati rice
- ¾ cup coconut milk

Directions:

1. Heat up a pan with the oil over medium- high heat, add the oil, onion, garlic, stevia, carrots, curry powder, cinnamon and ginger, stir, cook for 5 minutes and transfer to your slow cooker.
2. Add squash, stock and coconut milk, stir, cover and cook on Low for 4 hours.
3. Divide the butternut mix between plates and serve as a side dish.
4. Enjoy!

Nutrition: calories 200, fat 4, fiber 4, carbs 17, protein 3

Sausage Side Dish

Preparation time: 10 minutes

Cooking time: 2 hours

Servings: 12

Ingredients:

- 1 pound no-sugar, beef sausage, chopped
- 2 tablespoons olive oil
- ½ pound mushrooms, chopped
- 6 celery ribs, chopped
- 2 yellow onions, chopped
- 2 garlic cloves, minced
- 1 tablespoon sage, dried
- 1 cup low-sodium veggie stock
- 1 cup cranberries, dried
- ½ cup sunflower seeds, peeled
- 1 whole wheat bread loaf, cubed

Directions:

1. Heat up a pan with the oil over medium- high heat, add beef, stir and brown for a few minutes.
2. Add mushrooms, onion, celery, garlic and sage, stir, cook for a few more minutes and transfer to your slow cooker.
3. Add stock, cranberries, sunflower seeds and the bread cubes, cover and cook on High for 2 hours.
4. Stir the whole mix, divide between plates and serve as a side dish.
5. Enjoy!

Nutrition: calories 200, fat 3, fiber 6, carbs 13, protein 4

Easy Potatoes Mix

Preparation time: 10 minutes
Cooking time: 6 hours
Servings: 8
Ingredients:

- 16 baby red potatoes, halved
- 1 carrot, sliced
- 1 celery rib, chopped
- ¼ cup yellow onion, chopped
- 2 cups low-sodium chicken stock
- 1 tablespoon parsley, chopped
- A pinch of black pepper
- 1 garlic clove minced
- 2 tablespoons olive oil

Directions:

1. In your slow cooker, mix the potatoes with the carrot, celery, onion, stock, parsley, garlic, oil and black pepper, toss, cover and cook on Low for 6 hours.
2. Divide between plates and serve as a side dish.
3. Enjoy!

Nutrition: calories 114, fat 3, fiber 3, carbs 18, protein 4

Black-Eyed Peas Mix

Preparation time: 10 minutes
Cooking time: 5 hours
Servings: 12
Ingredients:

- 17 ounces black-eyed peas
- ½ cup sausage, chopped
- 1 yellow onion, chopped
- 1 sweet red pepper, chopped
- 1 jalapeno, chopped
- 2 garlic cloves minced
- ½ teaspoon cumin, ground
- A pinch of black pepper
- 6 cups water
- 2 tablespoons cilantro, chopped

Directions:

1. In your slow cooker, mix the peas with the sausage, onion, red pepper, jalapeno, garlic, cumin, black pepper, water and cilantro, cover and cook on Low for 5 hours.
2. Divide between plates and serve as a side dish.
3. Enjoy!

Nutrition: calories 170, fat 3, fiber 7, carbs 20, protein 13

Turmeric Endives

Preparation time: 10 minutes
Cooking time: 20 minutes
Servings: 4
Ingredients:

- 2 endives, halved lengthwise
- 2 tablespoons olive oil
- 1 teaspoon rosemary, dried
- ½ teaspoon turmeric powder
- A pinch of black pepper

Directions:

1. Mix the endives with the oil and the other ingredients in a baking pan, toss gently, and bake at 400 degrees F within 20 minutes. Serve as a side dish.

Nutrition:
Calories 64; Protein 0.2g; Carbohydrates 0.8g; Fat 7.1g; Fiber 0.6g; Sodium 3mg; Potassium 50mg

Parmesan Endives

Preparation time: 10 minutes
Cooking time: 20 minutes
Servings: 4
Ingredients:

- 4 endives, halved lengthwise
- 1 tablespoon lemon juice
- 1 tablespoon lemon zest, grated
- 2 tablespoons fat-free parmesan, grated
- 2 tablespoons olive oil
- A pinch of black pepper

Directions:

1. In a baking dish, combine the endives with the lemon juice and the other ingredients except for the parmesan and toss. Sprinkle the parmesan on top, bake the endives at 400 degrees F for 20 minutes, and serve.

Nutrition:
Calories 71; Protein 0.9g; Carbohydrates 2.2g; Fat 7.1g; Fiber 0.9g; Sodium 71mg; Potassium 88mg

Lemon Asparagus

Preparation time: 10 minutes

Cooking time: 20 minutes

Servings: 4

Ingredients:

- 1-pound asparagus, trimmed
- 2 tablespoons basil pesto
- 1 tablespoon lemon juice
- A pinch of black pepper
- 3 tablespoons olive oil
- 2 tablespoons cilantro, chopped

Directions:

1. Arrange the asparagus n a lined baking sheet, add the pesto and the other ingredients, toss, bake at 400 degrees F within 20 minutes. Serve as a side dish.

Nutrition:

Calories 114; Protein 2.6g; Carbohydrates 4.5g; Fat 10.7g; Fiber 2.4g; Sodium 3mg; Potassium 240mg

Lime Carrots

Preparation time: 10 minutes
Cooking time: 30 minutes
Servings: 4
Ingredients:

- 1-pound baby carrots, trimmed
- 1 tablespoon sweet paprika
- 1 teaspoon lime juice
- 3 tablespoons olive oil
- A pinch of black pepper
- 1 teaspoon sesame seeds

Directions:

1. Arrange the carrots on a lined baking sheet, add the paprika and the other ingredients except for the sesame seeds, toss, and bake at 400 degrees F within 30 minutes. Divide the carrots between plates, sprinkle sesame seeds on top and serve as a side dish.

Nutrition:
Calories 139; Protein 1.1g; Carbohydrates 10.5g; Fat 11.2g; 4g fiber; Sodium 89mg; Potassium 313mg

Garlic Potato Pan

Preparation time: 10 minutes

Cooking time: 1 hour

Servings: 8

Ingredients:

- 1-pound gold potatoes, peeled and cut into wedges
- 2 tablespoons olive oil
- 1 red onion, chopped
- 2 garlic cloves, minced
- 2 cups coconut cream
- 1 tablespoon thyme, chopped
- ¼ teaspoon nutmeg, ground
- ½ cup low-fat parmesan, grated

Directions:

1. Warm-up a pan with the oil over medium heat, put the onion plus the garlic, and sauté for 5 minutes. Add the potatoes and brown them for 5 minutes more.
2. Add the cream and the rest of the ingredients, toss gently, bring to a simmer and cook over medium heat within 40 minutes more. Divide the mix between plates and serve as a side dish.

Nutrition:

Calories 230; Protein 3.6g; Carbohydrates 14.3g; Fat 19.1g; Fiber 3.3g; Cholesterol 6mg; Sodium 105mg; Potassium 426mg

CHAPTER 8:

Vegetables

Cauliflower Pizza Crust

Preparation time: 15 minutes
Cooking time: 20 minutes
Servings: 6

Ingredients:

- 2 cups cauliflower, chopped
- 1 egg, whisked
- 1 teaspoon butter
- 1 teaspoon dried basil
- 1 teaspoon salt
- 6 oz Cheddar cheese, shredded
- 1 tablespoon heavy cream

Directions:

1. Place the cauliflower in the food processor and blend until you get cauliflower rice.
2. Then squeeze the juice from the cauliflower rice.
3. Line the baking tray with the parchment and then spread parchment with the butter.
4. Place the cauliflower rice in the tray in the shape of the pizza crust.
5. Bake the cauliflower pizza crust for 10 minutes at 365F.
6. Meanwhile, mix up together salt, shredded Cheddar cheese, heavy cream, and egg.
7. When the cauliflower crust is cooked, spread it with cheese mixture and flatten gently it.
8. Bake the meal for 10 minutes more at 375F.
9. When the pizza crust is cooked, cut it into 6 servings.

Nutrition: calories 147, fat 11.7, fiber 0.8, carbs 2.3, protein 8.7

Zucchini Ravioli

Preparation time: 20 minutes
Cooking time: 15 minutes
Servings: 4

Ingredients:

- 1 zucchini, trimmed
- 2 tablespoons ricotta cheese
- ½ cup spinach, chopped
- 1 teaspoon olive oil
- ½ teaspoon salt
- 1/3 cup marinara sauce
- 4 oz Parmesan, grated

Directions:

1. Slice the zucchini with the help of the peeler to get long slices.
2. Then take 4 zucchini slices and make the cross from them.
3. Repeat the same steps with all remaining zucchini slices.
4. After this, place chopped spinach in the skillet.
5. Add salt and olive oil. Mix up spinach and cook it for 5 minutes. Stir it from time to time.
6. After this, mix up spinach with ricotta and stir well.
7. Pour marinara sauce in the casserole dish.
8. Place the ricotta mixture in the center of every zucchini cross and fold up them.
9. Transfer zucchini balls -ravioli in the casserole to dish on the marinara sauce.
10. Sprinkle the zucchini ravioli over with grated Parmesan and transfer the casserole dish in the preheated to the 395F oven. Cook the meal for 15 minutes.

Nutrition: calories 141, fat 8.9, fiber 1.2, carbs 5.9, protein 11.1

Vegetable Crackers

Preparation time: 20 minutes
Cooking time: 20 minutes
Servings: 4

Ingredients:

- 1 cup cauliflower
- 1 tablespoon flax meal
- 1 teaspoon chia seeds
- 1 teaspoon ground cumin
- 1 teaspoon salt
- ½ teaspoon ground paprika
- 1 tablespoon rice flour
- 1 teaspoon nutritional yeast
- 1 cup water, for the steamer

Directions:

1. Chop the cauliflower roughly.
2. Pour water in the steamer and insert steamer rack. Place the cauliflower in the rack and close the lid.
3. Preheat the steamer and steam cauliflower for 5 minutes.
4. After this, place the vegetables in the food processor and blend well.
5. Transfer the blended cauliflower in the cheesecloth and squeeze the liquid from it.
6. Then transfer the cauliflower in the bowl.
7. Add all ingredients from the list above and mix up well.
8. Line the baking tray with the parchment and place cauliflower mixture over it.
9. Cover it with the second parchment sheet.
10. Roll up the cauliflower mixture into the rectangular.
11. Remove the upper parchment sheet and cut the cauliflower mixture into the crackers.
12. Transfer the tray in the preheated to the 365F oven.
13. Cook crackers for 15 minutes.
14. Chill the crackers well remove from the baking tray.

Nutrition: calories 35, fat 1.3, fiber 2.1, carbs 5.2, protein 1.8

Crunchy Okra Bites

Preparation time: 10 minutes
Cooking time: 12 minutes
Servings: 2
Ingredients:

- 1 cup okra, roughly sliced
- ¼ cup almond flour
- 1 tablespoon coconut flakes
- 1 teaspoon chili powder
- ½ teaspoon salt
- 3 eggs, whisked

Directions:

1. In the mixing bowl, mix up together almond flour, coconut flakes, chili powder, and salt.
2. Place the sliced okra into the whisked egg and mix up well.
3. Then coat every okra bite into the almond flour mixture.
4. Line the tray with the parchment.
5. Place the okra bites into the tray to make the okra layer.
6. Preheat the oven to 375F.
7. Place the tray with okra bites in the oven and cook for 12 minutes.
8. Chill the hot okra bites little before serving.

Nutrition: calories 147, fat 9.5, fiber 2.7, carbs 6.1, protein 10.3

Arugula-Tomato Salad

Preparation time: 15 minutes

Servings: 6

Ingredients:

- 2 cups arugula, chopped
- 1 cup lettuce, chopped
- ½ cup cherry tomatoes
- ¼ cup fresh basil
- 1 tablespoon olive oil
- ½ teaspoon chili flakes
- 5 oz Mozzarella cheese balls, cherry size

Directions:

1. Make the salad dressing: blend the fresh basil until smooth and add olive oil and chili flakes. Pulse the mixture for 5 seconds.
2. After this, place arugula and lettuce into the salad bowl.
3. Cut the cherry tomatoes into the halves and add in the salad bowl.
4. Then add Mozzarella cheese balls and shake the salad well.
5. Pour the salad dressing over the salad.

Nutrition: calories 93, fat 8.3, fiber 0.4, carbs 1.1, protein 4.5

Basil Bake

Preparation time: 15 minutes
Cooking time: 25 minutes
Servings: 4

Ingredients:

- ½ cup fresh basil
- 4 tablespoons coconut oil
- 1 zucchini, sliced
- 2 oz Parmesan, grated
- 1 tablespoon walnuts, chopped
- ½ teaspoon salt
- 2 tomatoes, sliced

Directions:

1. Melt coconut oil and transfer it in the blender.
2. Add fresh basil, walnuts, and salt. Blend the mixture until smooth. Add grated Parmesan and stir it. The pesto sauce is cooked.
3. Place the sliced zucchini and tomatoes into the casserole dish one-by-one.
4. Then top it with pesto sauce.
5. Cover the casserole dish with the foil and transfer in the oven.
6. Bake the meal for 25 minutes at 375F.
7. Then discard the foil and remove the basil bake from the oven.

Nutrition: calories 194, fat 18, fiber 1.5, carbs 4.8, protein 6.2

Roasted Bok Choy with Chili Sauce

Preparation time: 10 minutes

Cooking time: 10 minutes

Servings: 2

Ingredients:

- 8 oz bok choy
- 4 tablespoons chili sauce
- 2 tablespoons almond butter
- 1 teaspoon dried dill

Directions:

1. Slice bok choy into halves and place in the big bowl.
2. Add chili sauce and dried dill and mix up well.
3. Place the almond butter in the skillet and melt it.
4. Add the chili bok choy and roast it for 5 minutes from each side over the medium-low heat.
5. Gently transfer the cooked bok choy into the serving plates.

Nutrition: calories 117, fat 9.4, fiber 2.9, carbs 6.3, protein 5.4

Vegan Moussaka

Preparation time: 15 minutes
Cooking time: 35 minutes
Servings: 88
Ingredients:

- 2 eggplants, trimmed
- 1 white onion, chopped
- 1 garlic clove, diced
- ¼ cup tomatoes, crushed
- ½ teaspoon ground cinnamon
- 1 teaspoon salt
- 1 teaspoon ground black pepper
- 1 teaspoon ground paprika
- 2 tablespoons coconut oil
- 2 tablespoons ricotta cheese
- 1 oz Cheddar cheese, shredded
- 1 tablespoon heavy cream

Directions:

1. Place the coconut oil in the saucepan and melt it.
2. Meanwhile, chop the eggplants.
3. Place the eggplants and onion in the hot coconut oil. Add diced garlic.
4. Mix up the vegetables and cook them for 10 minutes or until they start to be soft.
5. Meanwhile, mix up together heavy cream, ricotta cheese, and shredded Cheddar cheese.
6. Transfer the roasted vegetables in the blender and blend for 3 minutes or until they are smooth.
7. After this, add all spices and crushed tomatoes, Blend the mixture 1 minute more.
8. Transfer the eggplant mixture in the casserole dish and flatten it well with the help of the spatula.
9. Place ricotta mixture over the eggplant mixture.
10. Bake moussaka for 20 minutes at the preheated to the 360F oven.
11. Chill the cooked meal for 10 minutes before serving.

Nutrition: calories 99, fat 5.9, fiber 5.5, carbs 10.4, protein 3

Cumin Fennel

Preparation time: 10 minutes
Cooking time: 15 minutes
Servings: 6

Ingredients:
- 1-pound fennel bulb
- 2 tablespoons butter, softened
- 1 tablespoon ground cumin
- 1 teaspoon salt
- ¼ teaspoon garlic powder

Directions:
1. Slice fennel bulb into the medium slices.
2. Line the baking tray with the baking paper.
3. Churn butter with the ground cumin, salt, and garlic powder.
4. Arrange the sliced fennel on the tray and spread it with the churned butter mixture.
5. Bake the fennel for 15 minutes at 360F.
6. When the fennel is cooked, it has a tender taste.

Nutrition: calories 62, fat 4.2, fiber 2.5, carbs 6, protein 1.2

Mushroom Tart

Preparation time: 15 minutes
Cooking time: 40 minutes
Servings: 8

Ingredients:

- 1 teaspoon baking powder
- ½ teaspoon salt
- 1 small egg, beaten
- 1 tablespoon coconut oil
- ½ cup almond flour
- 1 cup mushroom caps
- 1 tablespoon fresh dill, chopped
- 1 tablespoon butter
- 1 teaspoon ground turmeric
- 1 teaspoon ground paprika
- 2 oz Parmesan, grated
- ¼ cup heavy cream

Directions:

1. Make the tart dough: mix up together salt, egg baking powder, coconut oil, and almond flour. Knead the dough and roll it up into the pie crust.
2. Place the dough into the pie form.
3. Then arrange the mushrooms caps inside the pie form.
4. Sprinkle them with chopped dill, ground turmeric, paprika, and butter.
5. Then add Parmesan and pour it over with the heavy cream.
6. Transfer the tart in the oven.
7. Cook the mushroom tart for 40 minutes at 360F.
8. Chill the cooked tart till them room temperature and after this cut it into the servings.

Nutrition: calories 85, fat 7.5, fiber 0.5, carbs 1.9, protein 3.8

Cauliflower Cheese

Preparation time: 10 minutes

Cooking time: 25 minutes

Servings: 5

Ingredients:

- 2 cups cauliflower florets
- 1 cup organic almond milk
- ½ cup heavy cream
- 2 tablespoons coconut flour
- 1 teaspoon salt
- 6 oz Cheddar cheese, shredded
- 2 cups of water

Directions:

1. Bring water to boil, add cauliflower florets and boil them for 10 minutes.
2. Then drain water and transfer cauliflower florets in the baking dish.
3. Pour almond milk and heavy cream in the saucepan. Bring the liquid to boil.
4. Add salt and coconut flour.
5. Whisk the liquid very fast for 1 minute.
6. Then switch off the heat and add shredded cheese.
7. Leave the liquid until cheese is melted. Mix it up.
8. Pour cheese over the cauliflower florets.
9. Bake the cauliflower cheese for 15 minutes at 375F or until it starts bubbling.

Nutrition: calories 225, fat 17.1, fiber 3, carbs 7.7, protein 10.5

Spinach & Kale Salad

Preparation time: 10 minutes
Cooking time: 25 minutes
Servings: 4
Ingredients:

- 2 cups fresh spinach
- 1 cucumber, chopped
- 1 cup kale
- ¼ teaspoon salt
- ½ teaspoon ground black pepper
- 1 teaspoon flax seeds
- 1 bell pepper
- 2 tablespoons sesame oil
- 2 tablespoons lemon juice
- ½ cup lettuce

Directions:

1. Remove stems from kale.
2. Roughly chop kale, spinach, and lettuce and transfer greens in the salad bowl.
3. Slice bell pepper.
4. Add sliced bell pepper and chopped cucumber in the salad bowl too.
5. Then sprinkle the meal with salt, ground black pepper, lemon juice, and sesame oil.
6. Mix up a salad with the help of 2 forks.

Nutrition: calories 99, fat 7.3, fiber 1.7, carbs 8, protein 2

Cauliflower Anti Pasto

Preparation time: 10 minutes
Cooking time: 20 minutes
Servings: 4

Ingredients:

- 1 cup mushrooms, marinated, chopped
- 1 cup cauliflower
- 2 oz Swiss cheese, chopped
- 1 bell pepper, chopped
- 1 teaspoon dried oregano
- 1 tablespoon lemon juice
- 1 tablespoon olive oil
- ½ teaspoon dried cilantro
- 1 cup water, for the steamer

Directions:

1. Pour water in the steamer and insert trivet.
2. Place the cauliflower in the trivet and close the lid.
3. Steam the vegetable for 10 minutes totally -including preheating.
4. Preheat oven to 375F.
5. Place bell peppers in the tray and transfer in the oven.
6. Bake it for 5 minutes from each side.
7. Remove the cooked bell pepper from the oven, chill little and peel.
8. Then chop it roughly and put in the big bowl.
9. Remove the cauliflower from the steamer and cut it into the small florets.
10. Transfer the cauliflower in the zip log bag.
11. Add dried oregano, lemon juice, olive oil, and dried cilantro.
12. Shake the mixture well.
13. Remove the cauliflower from the zip log into the bowl with the bell pepper.
14. Add chopped Swiss cheese and marinated mushrooms.
15. Mix up antipasto well.

Nutrition: calories 105, fat 7.7, fiber 1.4, carbs 5.2, protein 5.2

Sour Sweet Bok Choy

Preparation time: 7 minutes
Cooking time: 12 minutes
Servings: 1

Ingredients:

- 6 oz bok choy, sliced
- 1 teaspoon Erythritol
- 1 teaspoon lime juice
- ¼ teaspoon ground paprika
- 1 tablespoon water
- 1 teaspoon apple cider vinegar
- 1 tablespoon almond butter

Directions:

1. Put almond butter in the skillet and melt it.
2. Add sliced bok choy and roast it for 3 minutes from each side.
3. Meanwhile, whisk together Erythritol, lime juice, ground paprika, water, and apple cider vinegar.
4. When the bok choy is roasted from both sides sprinkle it with Erythritol mixture and mix up with the help of a spatula.
5. Bring to boil the meal and switch off the heat.
6. Let bok choy rest for 5 minutes.

Nutrition: calories 124, fat 9.4, fiber 3.5, carbs 7.4, protein 6

Celery Rosti

Preparation time: 10 minutes
Cooking time: 10 minutes
Servings: 4

Ingredients:

- 8 oz celery root, peeled
- 1/3 onion, diced
- 1 teaspoon olive oil
- ½ teaspoon ground black pepper
- 2 oz Parmesan, grated
- ¼ teaspoon ground turmeric

Directions:

1. Put the diced onion in the skillet. Add olive oil and cook it until translucent.
2. Meanwhile, grated celery root and mix it up with ground black pepper, ground turmeric, and Parmesan.
3. When the mixture is homogenous, add it in the skillet.
4. Mix up well.
5. Then press the celery root mixture with the help of the spatula to get the shape of the pancake.
6. Close the lid and cook celery rosti for 6 minutes or until it is light brown.

Nutrition: calories 84, fat 4.4, fiber 1.3, carbs 6.9, protein 5.5

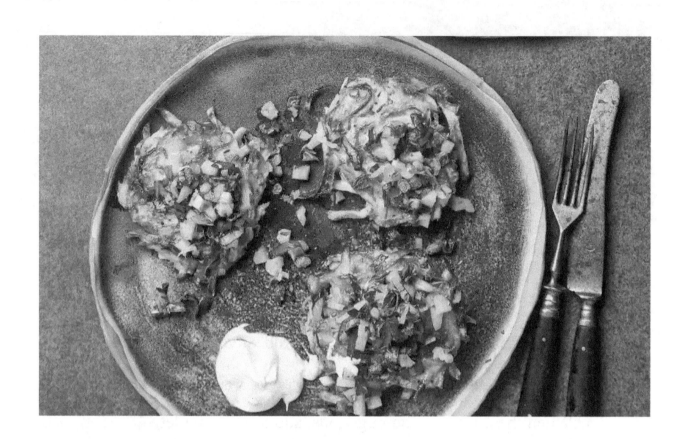

Garlic Snap Peas

Preparation time: 5 minutes
Cooking time: 10 minutes
Servings: 3
Ingredients:

- 1 cup snap peas
- 1 teaspoon Erythritol
- 1 teaspoon avocado oil
- ¼ teaspoon cayenne pepper
- ½ teaspoon garlic powder
- ¾ teaspoon garlic, diced

Directions:

1. Pour avocado oil in the skillet.
2. Add diced garlic and cook it for 1 minute over the medium heat.
3. Sprinkle it with garlic powder, cayenne pepper, and Erythritol.
4. Then add snap peas and mix up well.
5. Cook the snap peas for 9 minutes. Stir it all the time.
6. The cooked snap peas should be tender and crispy.

Nutrition: calories 44, fat 0.4, fiber 2.6, carbs 7.7, protein 2.8

Sheet Pan Rosemary Mushrooms

Preparation time: 10 minutes

Cooking time: 15 minutes

Servings: 2

Ingredients:

- 1 cup mushrooms
- 1 teaspoon minced rosemary
- ½ teaspoon of sea salt
- 1 tablespoon sesame oil

Directions:

- Line the baking tray with baking paper.
- Slice the mushrooms roughly and put them in the baking tray.
- Sprinkle mushrooms with minced rosemary, sea salt, and sesame oil.
- Mix up the vegetables well with the help of the hand palms.
- Preheat the oven to 360F.
- Cook mushrooms for 15 minutes.

Nutrition: calories 70, fat 7, fiber 0.6, carbs 1.5, protein 1.1

Buttered Sprouts

Preparation time: 7 minutes
Cooking time: 20 minutes
Servings: 4

Ingredients:

- 10 oz Brussels sprouts
- 2 oz prosciutto
- 3 teaspoons butter
- 1 cup of water
- 1 teaspoon salt

Directions:

1. Chop prosciutto and place in the saucepan.
2. Roast it until it starts to be crispy.
3. Then add water and Brussels sprouts.
4. Bring the mixture to boil and close the lid.
5. Boil the vegetables for 15 minutes.
6. After this, drain ½ part of all liquid and add butter.
7. Mix it up until the butter is melted and bring the meal to boil one more time in the butter liquid.
8. Serve buttered sprouts with the butter liquid.

Nutrition: calories 76, fat 3.9, fiber 2.7, carbs 6.7, protein 5.4

Bacon Cabbage Slices

Preparation time: 10 minutes

Cooking time: 15 minutes

Servings: 4

Ingredients:

- 10 oz white cabbage
- 4 oz bacon, sliced
- ½ teaspoon ground black pepper
- 1 teaspoon butter
- ½ teaspoon salt

Directions:

1. Slice the cabbage into medium slices and rub with butter.
2. Sprinkle the bacon slices with ground black pepper and salt.
3. Wrap every cabbage slice into the bacon and transfer in the tray.
4. Cook the cabbage slices in the oven at 370F for 15 minutes. You can flip the cabbage slices onto another side during cooking.

Nutrition: calories 180, fat 12.9, fiber 1.8, carbs 4.7, protein 11.5

Lemon Onion Mash

Preparation time: 15 minutes
Cooking time: 15 minutes
Servings: 4

Ingredients:

- 2 white onions
- 4 oz cauliflower
- ¼ cup heavy cream
- 4 oz Cheddar cheese, shredded
- ½ teaspoon Pink salt
- 1 teaspoon white pepper
- ½ teaspoon lemon zest
- 1 teaspoon lemon juice
- 1 teaspoon butter

Directions:

1. Peel the onion and grind it.
2. Put grinded onion and butter in the saucepan.
3. Blend cauliflower until you get cauliflower rice.
4. Add cauliflower rice in the saucepan too.
5. Add pink salt, white pepper, lemon zest, and lemon juice. Stir it.
6. Close the lid and cook the mass for 5 minutes over the medium heat.
7. Then add shredded Cheddar cheese and heavy cream.
8. Mix up well and stir it until cheese is melted.
9. Close the lid and simmer mash for 5 minutes more over the low heat.
10. Switch off the heat and close the lid.
11. Let the lemon onion mash chill for 10 minutes.

Nutrition: calories 179, fat 13.3, fiber 2.1, carbs 7.6, protein 8.5

Chopped Ragu

Preparation time: 10 minutes
Cooking time: 25 minutes
Servings: 5

Ingredients:

- 1 bell pepper, chopped
- 2 oz green beans, chopped
- 1 oz bok choy, chopped
- 2 oz collard greens, chopped
- ½ white onion, chopped
- 3 oz kale, chopped
- 2 oz jicama, chopped
- 3 oz asparagus
- ½ cup of coconut milk
- 1/3 cup water
- 1 teaspoon salt
- ½ teaspoon ground black pepper
- ½ teaspoon cayenne pepper
- 1 teaspoon marinara sauce

Directions:

1. Take the big pan and add water inside.
2. Bring water to boil and add chopped bell pepper, green beans, bok choy, collard greens, onion, kale, jicama, and asparagus.
3. Then add salt, ground black pepper, cayenne pepper, and marinara sauce.
4. Add coconut milk and carefully stir the vegetable ragu.
5. Preheat the oven to 365F.
6. Close the lid of the pan.
7. Transfer the pan in the preheated oven and bake ragu for 25 minutes.

8. When the ragu is cooked, remove it from the oven and remove the lid.
9. Don't stir ragu anymore!
10. If ragu will chill for 10-15 minutes, you will get the most delicious taste of ragu.

Nutrition: calories 93, fat 6, fiber 3.2, carbs 9.5, protein 2.5

CHAPTER 9:

EGGS AND DAIRY RECIPES

Eggtastic Smoothie

Servings: 1
Preparation time: 10 minutes
Cooking time: 5 minutes

Ingredients

- 2 tablespoons cream cheese
- 2 raw eggs
- 1 tablespoon vanilla extract
- ¼ cup heavy cream
- 3 ice cubes

Directions

1. Put all the ingredients in a blender and blend until smooth.
2. Pour into 1 glass and immediately serve.

Nutrition:

Calories   337
Total Fat 26.8g
Saturated Fat 14g
Cholesterol 390mg   1
Sodium 195mg
Total Carbohydrate 3.7g
Dietary Fiber 0g
Total Sugars 2.4g Protein 13.2g

Eggs and Bacon

Servings: 12
Preparation time: 35 mins
Cooking time: 15 minutes

Ingredients

- ½ teaspoon dried organic thyme
- 7 oz full fat cream cheese
- ½ cup parmesan cheese, shredded
- 24 organic bacon slices
- 12 hard cooked organic large eggs, peeled, yolks removed and sliced lengthwise

Directions

1. Preheat the oven to 3900F and lightly grease a baking dish.
2. Mix together thyme and cream cheese in a bowl.
3. Fill the egg white halves with the thyme mixture and close with the other egg white halves.
4. Wrap each egg tightly with 2 bacon slices and arrange on the baking dish.
5. Transfer to the oven and bake for about 25 minutes.
6. Remove from the oven to serve warm.

Nutrition:

Calories   340 Total Fat 25.9g
Saturated Fat 10.5g
Cholesterol 239mg
Sodium 1219mg
Total Carbohydrate 2.1g
Dietary Fiber 0.3g
Total Sugars 1.2g
Protein 23.9g

Moroccan-Inspired Tagine with Chickpeas & Vegetables

Preparation time: 15 minutes
Cooking time: 45 minutes
Servings: 3
Ingredients:

- 2 teaspoons olive oil
- 1 cup chopped carrots
- ½ cup finely chopped onion
- 1 sweet potato, diced
- 1 cup low-sodium vegetable broth
- ¼ teaspoon ground cinnamon
- 1/8 teaspoon salt
- 1½ cups chopped bell peppers, any color
- 3 ripe plum tomatoes, chopped
- 1 tablespoon tomato paste
- 1 garlic clove, pressed or minced
- 1 (15-ounce) can chickpeas, drained and rinsed
- ½ cup chopped dried apricots
- 1 teaspoon curry powder
- ½ teaspoon paprika
- ½ teaspoon turmeric

Directions:

1. Warm-up oil over medium heat in a large Dutch oven or saucepan. Add the carrots and onion and cook until the onion is translucent about 4 minutes. Add the sweet potato, broth, cinnamon, and salt and cook for 5 to 6 minutes, until the broth is slightly reduced.
2. Add the peppers, tomatoes, tomato paste, and garlic. Stir and cook for another 5 minutes. Add the chickpeas, apricots, curry powder, paprika, and turmeric to the pot. Bring all to a boil, then reduce the heat to low, cover, simmer for about 30 minutes, and serve.

Nutrition:
Calories: 469; Fat: 9g; Carbohydrates: 88g; Protein: 16g; Sodium: 256mg

Spaghetti Squash with Maple Glaze & Tofu Crumbles

Preparation time: 15 minutes

Cooking time: 22 minutes

Servings: 3

Ingredients:

- 2 ounces firm tofu, well-drained
- 1 small spaghetti squash, halved lengthwise
- 2½ teaspoons olive oil, divided
- 1/8 teaspoon salt
- ½ cup chopped onion
- 1 teaspoon dried rosemary
- ¼ cup dry white wine
- 2 tablespoons maple syrup
- ½ teaspoon garlic powder
- ¼ cup shredded Gruyere cheese

Directions:

1. Put the tofu in a large mesh colander and place over a large bowl to drain. Score the squash using a paring knife so the steam can vent while it cooks. Place the squash in a medium microwave-safe dish and microwave on high for 5 minutes. Remove the squash from the microwave and allow it to cool.

2. Cut the cooled squash in half on a cutting board. Remove the seeds, then put the squash halves into a 9-by-11-inch baking dish.

3. Drizzle the squash with half a teaspoon of olive oil and season it with the salt, then wrap it using wax paper and put it back in the microwave for 5 more minutes on high. Once it's cooked, scrape the squash strands with a fork into a small bowl and cover it to keep it warm.

4. While the squash is cooking, heat 1 teaspoon of oil in a large skillet over medium-high heat. Put the onion and sauté for within minutes. Add the rosemary and stir for 1 minute, until fragrant.

5. Put the rest of the oil in the same skillet. Crumble the tofu into the skillet, stir fry until lightly browned, about 4 minutes, and transfer it to a small bowl.

6. Add the wine, maple syrup, and garlic powder to the skillet and stir to combine. Cook for 2 minutes until slightly reduced and thickened. Remove from the heat. Evenly divide the squash between two plates,

then top it with the tofu mixture. Drizzle the maple glaze over the top, then add the grated cheese.

Nutrition:

Calories: 330; Fat: 15g; Carbohydrates: 36g; Fiber: 5g; Protein: 12g; Sodium: 326mg; Potassium: 474mg

Stuffed Tex-Mex Baked Potatoes

Preparation time: 15 minutes
Cooking time: 45 minutes
Servings: 2
Ingredients:

- 2 large Idaho potatoes
- ½ cup black beans, rinsed and drained
- ¼ cup store-bought salsa
- 1 avocado, diced
- 1 teaspoon freshly squeezed lime juice
- ½ cup nonfat plain Greek yogurt
- ¼ teaspoon reduced-sodium taco seasoning
- ¼ cup shredded sharp cheddar cheese

Directions:

1. Preheat the oven to 400°F. Scrub the potatoes, then slice an "X" into the top of each using a paring knife. Put the potatoes on the oven rack, then bake for 45 minutes until they are tender.
2. In a small bowl, stir the beans and salsa and set aside. In another small bowl, mix the avocado and lime juice and set aside. In a third small bowl, stir the yogurt and the taco seasoning until well blended.
3. When the potatoes are baked, carefully open them up. Top each potato with the bean and salsa mixture, avocado, seasoned yogurt, and cheddar cheese, evenly dividing each component, and serve.

Nutrition:
Calories: 624; Fat: 21g; Carbohydrates: 91g; Fiber: 21g; Protein: 24g; Sodium: 366mg; Potassium: 2134mg

Lentil-Stuffed Zucchini Boats

Preparation time: 15 minutes
Cooking time: 45 minutes
Servings: 2
Ingredients:

- 2 medium zucchinis, halved lengthwise and seeded
- 2¼ cups water, divided
- 1 cup green or red lentils, dried & rinsed
- 2 teaspoons olive oil
- 1/3 cup diced onion
- 2 tablespoons tomato paste
- ½ teaspoon oregano
- ¼ teaspoon garlic powder
- Pinch salt
- ¼ cup grated part-skim mozzarella cheese

Directions:

1. Preheat the oven to 375°F. Line a baking sheet with parchment paper. Place the zucchini, hollow sides up, on the baking sheet, and set aside.
2. Boil 2 cups of water to a boil over high heat in a medium saucepan and add the lentils. Lower the heat, then simmer within 20 to 25 minutes. Drain and set aside.
3. Heat-up the olive oil in a medium skillet over medium-low heat. Sauté the onions until they are translucent, about 4 minutes. Lower the heat and add the cooked lentils, tomato paste, oregano, garlic powder, and salt.
4. Add the last quarter cup of water and simmer for 3 minutes, until the liquid reduces and forms a sauce. Remove from heat.
5. Stuff each zucchini half with the lentil mixture, dividing it evenly, and top with cheese, bake for 25 minutes and serve. The zucchini should be fork-tender, and the cheese should be melted.

Nutrition:
Calories: 479; Fat: 9g; Carbohydrates: 74g; Fiber: 14g; Protein: 31g; Sodium: 206mg; Potassium: 1389mg

Baked Eggplant Parmesan

Preparation time: 15 minutes
Cooking time: 35 minutes
Servings: 4
Ingredients:
- 1 small to medium eggplant, cut into ¼-inch slices
- ½ teaspoon salt-free Italian seasoning blend
- 1 tablespoon olive oil
- ¼ cup diced onion
- ½ cup diced yellow or red bell pepper
- 2 garlic cloves, pressed or minced
- 1 (8-ounce) can tomato sauce
- 3 ounces fresh mozzarella, cut into 6 pieces
- 1 tablespoon grated Parmesan cheese, divided
- 5 to 6 fresh basil leaves, chopped

Directions:
1. Preheat an oven-style air fryer to 400°F.
2. Working in two batches, place the eggplant slices onto the air-fryer tray and sprinkle them with Italian seasoning. Bake for 7 minutes. Repeat with the remaining slices, then set them aside on a plate.
3. In a medium skillet, heat the oil over medium heat and sauté the onion and peppers until softened about 5 minutes. Add the garlic and sauté for 1 to 2 more minutes. Add the tomato sauce and stir to combine. Remove the sauce from the heat.
4. Spray a 9-by-6-inch casserole dish with cooking spray. Spread one-third of the sauce into the bottom of the dish. Layer eggplant slices onto the sauce. Sprinkle with half of the Parmesan cheese.
5. Continue layering the sauce and eggplant, ending with the sauce. Place the mozzarella pieces on the top. Sprinkle the remaining Parmesan evenly over the entire dish. Bake in the oven for 20 minutes. Garnish with fresh basil, cut into four servings, and serve.

Nutrition:
Calories: 213; Fat: 12g; Carbohydrates: 20g; Fiber: 7g; Protein: 10g; Sodium: 222mg; Potassium: 763mg

Cheesy Ham Souffle

Servings: 4

Preparation time: 30 minutes

Cooking time: 15 minutes

Ingredients

- ½ cup heavy cream
- 1 cup cheddar cheese, shredded
- 6 large eggs
- Salt and black pepper, to taste
- 6 ounces ham, diced

Directions

1. Preheat the oven to 3750F and lightly grease ramekins.
2. Whisk together ham with all other ingredients in a bowl.
3. Mix well and pour the mixture into the ramekins.
4. Transfer to the oven and bake for about 20 minutes.
5. Remove from the oven and slightly cool before serving.

Nutrition:

Calories   342

Total Fat 26g

Saturated Fat 13g

Cholesterol 353mg   1

Sodium 841mg

Total Carbohydrate 3g

Dietary Fiber 0.6g

Total Sugars 0

Protein 23.8g

Mushroom and Cheese Scrambled Eggs

Servings: 4
Preparation time: 20 mins
Cooking time: 15 minutes

Ingredients

- 8 eggs
- 4 tablespoons butter
- 4 tablespoons parmesan cheese, shredded
- 1 cup fresh mushrooms, finely chopped
- Salt and black pepper, to taste

Directions

1. Whisk together eggs with salt and black pepper in a bowl until well combined.
2. Heat butter in a nonstick pan and stir in the whisked eggs.
3. Cook for about 4 minutes and add mushrooms and parmesan cheese.
4. Cook for about 6 minutes, occasionally stirring and dish out to serve.

Nutrition:

Calories   265 Total Fat 22.6g
Saturated Fat 11.5g   Cholesterol 365mg   1
Sodium 304mg   Total Carbohydrate 1.7g
Dietary Fiber 0.2g
Total Sugars 1g
Protein 15.1g

Red Pepper Frittata

Servings: 3
Preparation time: 15 mins
Cooking time: 15 minutes

Ingredients

- 6 large eggs
- 2 red peppers, chopped
- Salt and black pepper, to taste
- 1¼ cups mozzarella cheese, shredded
- 3 tablespoons olive oil

Directions

1. Whisk together the eggs in a medium bowl and add red peppers, mozzarella cheese, salt and black pepper.
2. Heat olive oil over medium high heat in an ovenproof skillet and pour in the egg mixture.
3. Lift the mixture with a spatula to let the eggs run under.
4. Cook for about 5 minutes, stirring well and dish out onto a platter to serve.

Nutrition:

Calories 308 Total Fat 26.2g
Saturated Fat 6.4g Cholesterol 378mg 1
Sodium 214mg Total Carbohydrate 3.9g
Dietary Fiber 0.5g
Total Sugars 2.4g
Protein 16.5g

Cream Cheese Pancakes

Servings: 4

Preparation time: 25 mins

Cooking time: 15 minutes

Ingredients

- ½ cup almond flour
- 2 scoops Stevia
- ½ teaspoon cinnamon
- 2 eggs
- 2 oz cream cheese

Directions

1. Put all the ingredients in a blender and blend until smooth.
2. Dish out the mixture to a medium bowl and set aside.
3. Heat butter in a skillet over medium heat and add one quarter of the mixture.
4. Spread the mixture and cook for about 4 minutes on both sides until golden brown.
5. Repeat with rest of the mixture in batches and serve warm.

Nutrition:

Calories   166

Total Fat 13.8g

Saturated Fat 4.3g

Cholesterol 97mg

Sodium 78mg

Total Carbohydrate 3.8g

Dietary Fiber 1.7g

Total Sugars 0.2g

Protein 6.9g

Spicy Chorizo Baked Eggs

Servings: 4

Preparation time: 40 mins

Cooking time: 15 minutes

Ingredients

- 5 large eggs
- 3 ounces ground chorizo sausage
- ¾ cup pepper jack cheese, shredded
- Salt and paprika, to taste
- 1 small avocado, chopped

Directions

Preheat the oven to 4000F.

1. Heat a nonstick oven safe skillet and add chorizo.
2. Cook for about 8 minutes and dish into a bowl.
3. Break the eggs in the skillet and season with salt and paprika.
4. Add cooked chorizo and avocado and cook for about 2 minutes.
5. Top with pepper jack cheese and transfer to the oven.
6. Bake for about 20 minutes and remove from the oven to serve.

Nutrition:

Calories   334

Total Fat 28.3g

Saturated Fat 10.3g

Cholesterol 269mg

Sodium 400mg

Total Carbohydrate 5.7g

Dietary Fiber 3.6g

Total Sugars 0.8g

Protein 16.9g

Cheesy Taco Pie

Servings: 6
Preparation time: 45 minutes
Cooking time: 15 minutes

Ingredients

- 1 tablespoon garlic powder
- 1 pound ground beef
- 6 large eggs
- Salt and chili powder, to taste
- 1 cup cheddar cheese, shredded

Directions

1. Preheat the oven to 3500F and lightly grease a pie plate.
2. Heat a large nonstick skillet and add beef, garlic powder, salt and chili powder.
3. Cook for about 6 minutes over medium low heat and transfer to the pie plate.
4. Top with cheddar cheese and transfer to the oven.
5. Bake for about 30 minutes and remove from the oven to serve hot.

Nutrition:

Calories 294
Total Fat 16g
Saturated Fat 7.3g
Cholesterol 273mg
Sodium 241mg
Total Carbohydrate 1.9g
Dietary Fiber 0.3g
Total Sugars 0.9g
Protein 34.2g

Sausage Egg Casserole

Servings: 8
Preparation time: 40 mins
Cooking time: 15 minutes

Ingredients

- 1 cup almond milk, unsweetened
- 6 large eggs
- Salt and black pepper, to taste
- 2 cups cheddar cheese, shredded
- 1 pound ground pork sausage, cooked

Directions

1. Preheat the oven to 3500F and lightly grease a casserole dish.
2. Whisk together eggs with almond milk, salt and black pepper in a bowl.
3. Put the cooked sausages in the casserole dish and top with the egg mixture and cheddar cheese.
4. Transfer to the oven and bake for about 30 minutes.
5. Remove from the oven and serve hot.

Nutrition:

Calories   429
Total Fat 36.3g
Saturated Fat 18.6g
Cholesterol 217mg
Sodium 657mg
Total Carbohydrate 2.3g
Dietary Fiber 0.7g
Total Sugars 1.4g
Protein 23.5g

Egg Bites

Servings: 8
Preparation time: 25 mins
Cooking time: 15 minutes

Ingredients

- 12 large eggs
- 1 -8-ounce package cream cheese, softened
- 8 slices bacon, cooked and crumbled
- 1 cup gruyere cheese, shredded
- Salt and paprika, to taste

Directions

1. Put eggs, cream cheese, salt and paprika in a blender and blend until smooth.
2. Grease 8 egg poaching cups lightly with cooking spray and put half the gruyere cheese, bacon and egg mixture in them.
3. Put the cups in a large saucepan with boiling water and cover the lid.
4. Lower the heat and cook for about 10 minutes.
5. Dish out the eggs into a serving dish and slice to serve.

Nutrition:

Calories 365
Total Fat 29.7g
Saturated Fat 13.7g
Cholesterol 346mg 1
Sodium 673mg
Total Carbohydrate 1.7g
Dietary Fiber 0g
Total Sugars 0.7g
Protein 22.6g

Chorizo and Eggs

Servings: 2
Preparation time: 20 mins
Cooking time: 15 minutes

Ingredients

- ½ small yellow onion, chopped
- 1 teaspoon olive oil
- 2 -3-ounce chorizo sausages
- Salt and black pepper, to taste
- 4 eggs

Directions

1. Open the sausage casings and dish the meat into a bowl.
2. Heat olive oil over medium high heat in a large skillet and add onions.
3. Sauté for about 3 minutes and stir in the chorizo sausage.
4. Cook for about 4 minutes and add eggs, salt and black pepper.
5. Whisk well and cook for about 3 minutes.
6. Dish into a bowl and serve warm.

Nutrition:

Calories   270 Total Fat 21.8g
Saturated Fat 7.6g   Cholesterol 201mg
Sodium 587mg
Total Carbohydrate 2g
Dietary Fiber 0.2g
Total Sugars 0.7g
Protein 15.9g

Egg in the Avocado

Servings: 6
Preparation time: 25 mins
Cooking time: 15 minutes

Ingredients

- 3 medium avocados, cut in half, pitted, skin on
- 1 teaspoon garlic powder
- ¼ cup parmesan cheese, grated
- 6 medium eggs
- Sea salt and black pepper, to taste

Directions

1. Preheat the oven to 3500F and grease 6 muffin tins.
2. Put the avocado half in each muffin tin and season with garlic powder, sea salt, and black pepper.
3. Break 1 egg into each avocado and top with the parmesan cheese.
4. Transfer into the oven and bake for about 15 minutes.
5. Remove from the oven and serve warm.

Nutrition:

Calories 107 Total Fat 7.9g
Saturated Fat 2.5g   Cholesterol 167mg
Sodium 105mg   Total Carbohydrate 2.4g
Dietary Fiber 1.6g Total Sugars 0.5g
Protein 7.6g

Egg, Bacon and Cheese Cups

Servings: 6

Preparation time: 30 mins

Cooking time: 15 minutes

Ingredients

- ¼ cup frozen spinach, thawed and drained
- 6 large eggs
- 6 strips bacon
- Salt and black pepper, to taste
- ¼ cup sharp cheddar cheese

Directions

1. Preheat the oven to 4000and grease 6 muffin cups.
2. Whisk together eggs, spinach, salt and black pepper in a bowl.
3. Put the bacon slices in the muffin cups and pour in the egg spinach mixture.
4. Top with sharp cheddar cheese and transfer to the oven.
5. Bake for 15 minutes and remove from the oven to serve warm.

Nutrition:

Calories   194

Total Fat 14.5g

Saturated Fat 5.2g

Cholesterol 212mg

Sodium 539mg

Total Carbohydrate 0.8g

Dietary Fiber 0g

Total Sugars 0.4g

Protein 14.5g

Steak and Eggs

Servings: 4

Preparation time: 25 mins

Cooking time: 15 minutes

Ingredients

- 6 eggs
- 2 tablespoons butter
- 8 oz. sirloin steak
- Salt and black pepper, to taste
- ½ avocado, sliced

Directions

1. Heat butter in a pan on medium heat and fry the eggs.
2. Season with salt and black pepper and dish out onto a plate.
3. Cook the sirloin steak in another pan until desired doneness and slice into bite sized strips.
4. Season with salt and black pepper and dish out alongside the eggs.
5. Put the avocados with the eggs and steaks and serve.

Nutrition:

Calories   302

Total Fat 20.8g

Saturated Fat 8.1g

Cholesterol 311mg   1

Sodium 172mg

Total Carbohydrate 2.7g

Dietary Fiber 1.7g

Total Sugars 0.6g

Protein 26g

Butter Coffee

Servings: 4
Preparation time: 20 mins
Cooking time: 15 minutes

Ingredients

- ½ cup coconut milk
- ½ cup water
- 2 tablespoons coffee
- 1 tablespoon coconut oil
- 1 tablespoon grass fed butter

Directions

1. Heat water in a saucepan and add coffee.
2. Simmer for about 3 minutes and add coconut milk.
3. Simmer for another 3 minutes and allow to cool down.
4. Transfer to a blender along with coconut oil and butter.

5. Pour into a mug and serve immediately.

Nutrition:

   Calories   111 Total Fat 11.9g

   Saturated Fat 10.3g   Cholesterol 4mg

   Sodium 18mg

   Total Carbohydrate 1.7g

   Dietary Fiber 0.7g Total Sugars 1g

   Protein 0.7g

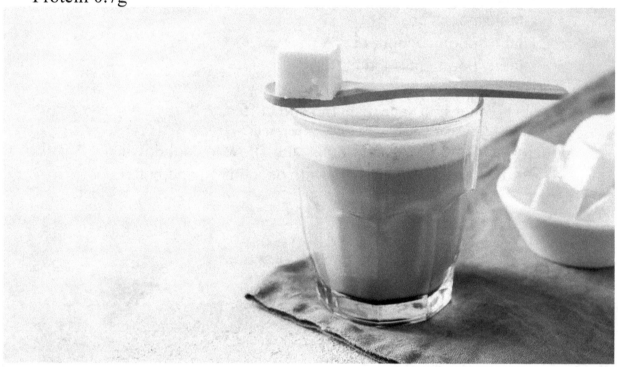

California Chicken Omelet

Servings: 1
Preparation time: 20 mins
Cooking time: 15 minutes

Ingredients

- 2 bacon slices, cooked and chopped
- 2 eggs
- 1 oz. deli cut chicken
- 3 tablespoons avocado mayonnaise
- 1 Campari tomato

Directions

1. Whisk together eggs in a bowl and pour into a nonstick pan.
2. Season with salt and black pepper and cook for about 5 minutes.
3. Add chicken, bacon, tomato and avocado mayonnaise and cover with lid.
4. Cook for 5 more minutes on medium low heat and dish out to serve hot.

Nutrition:

Calories   208
Total Fat 15g
Saturated Fat 4.5g
Cholesterol 189mg
Sodium 658mg
Total Carbohydrate 3g
Dietary Fiber 1.1g
Total Sugars 0.9g
Protein 15.3g

Eggs Oopsie Rolls

Servings: 3

Preparation time: 25 mins

Cooking time: 15 minutes

Ingredients

- 3 oz cream cheese
- 3 large eggs, separated
- 1/8 teaspoon cream of tartar
- 1 scoop stevia
- 1/8 teaspoon salt

Directions

1. Preheat oven to 3000F and line a cookie sheet with parchment paper.
2. Beat the egg whites with cream of tartar until soft peaks form.
3. Mix together egg yolks, salt and cream cheese in a bowl.
4. Combine the egg yolk and egg white mixtures and spoon them onto the cookie sheet.
5. Transfer to the oven and bake for about 40 minutes.
6. Remove from the oven and serve warm.

Nutrition:

Calories 171 Total Fat 14.9g

Saturated Fat 7.8g

Cholesterol 217mg

Sodium 251mg

Total Carbohydrate 1.2g

Dietary Fiber 0g

Total Sugars 0.5g

Protein 8.4g

Easy Blender Pancakes

Servings: 2
Preparation time: 25 mins
Cooking time: 15 minutes

Ingredients

- 2 eggs
- 2 oz. cream cheese
- 1 scoop Isopure Protein Powder
- 1 pinch salt
- 1 dash cinnamon

Directions

1. Mix together eggs with cream cheese, protein powder, salt and cinnamon in a bowl.
2. Transfer to a blender and blend until smooth.
3. Heat a nonstick pan and pour quarter of the mixture.
4. Cook for about 2 minutes on each side and dish out.
5. Repeat with the remaining mixture and dish out in a platter to serve warm.

Nutrition:

Calories   215 Total Fat 14.5g
Saturated Fat 7.7g   Cholesterol 196mg
Sodium 308mg   Total Carbohydrate 1.2g
Dietary Fiber 0.1g Total Sugars 0.4g
Protein 20.2g

Shakshuka

Servings: 2
Preparation time: 25 mins
Cooking time: 15 minutes

Ingredients

- 1 chili pepper, chopped
- 1 cup marinara sauce
- 4 eggs
- Salt and black pepper, to taste
- 1 oz. feta cheese

Directions

1. Preheat the oven to 3900F.
2. Heat a small oven proof skillet on medium heat and add marinara sauce and chili pepper.
3. Cook for about 5 minutes and stir in the eggs.
4. Season with salt and black pepper and top with feta cheese.
5. Transfer into the oven and bake for about 10 minutes.
6. Remove from the oven and serve hot shakshuka.

Nutrition:

Calories 273 Total Fat 15.1g
Saturated Fat 5.7g Cholesterol 342mg 1
Sodium 794mg Total Carbohydrate 18.7g
Dietary Fiber 3.3g
Total Sugars 12.4g
Protein 15.4g

Rooibos Tea Latte

Servings: 1
Preparation time: 20 mins
Cooking time: 15 minutes

Ingredients

- 2 bags rooibos tea
- 1 cup water
- 1 tablespoon grass fed butter
- 1 scoop collagen peptides
- ¼ cup full fat canned coconut milk

Directions

1. Put the tea bags in boiling water and steep for about 5 minutes.
2. Discard the tea bags and stir in butter and coconut milk.
3. Pour this mixture into a blender and blend until smooth.
4. Add collagen to the blender and blend on low speed until incorporated.
5. Pour into a mug to serve hot or chilled as desired.

Nutrition:

Calories 283
Total Fat 23.5g
Saturated Fat 18.3g
Cholesterol 31mg
Sodium 21mg
Total Carbohydrate 3.4g
Dietary Fiber 0g
Total Sugars 2.4g
Protein 15g

Feta and Pesto Omelet

Servings: 3
Preparation time: 10 mins
Cooking time: 15 minutes

Ingredients

- 3 eggs
- 2 tablespoons butter
- 1 oz. feta cheese
- Salt and black pepper, to taste
- 1 tablespoon pesto

Directions

1. Heat butter in a pan and allow it to melt.
2. Whisk together eggs in a bowl and pour into the pan.
3. Cook for about 3 minutes until done and add feta cheese and pesto.
4. Season with salt and black pepper and fold it over.
5. Cook for another 5 minutes until the feta cheese is melted and dish out onto a platter to serve.

Nutrition:

Calories   178
Total Fat 16.2g
Saturated Fat 8.1g
Cholesterol 194mg
Sodium 253mg
Total Carbohydrate 1.1g
Dietary Fiber 0.1g
Total Sugars 1.1g
Protein 7.5g

Eggs Benedict

Servings: 2
Preparation time: 25 mins
Cooking time: 15 minutes

Ingredients

- 4 oopsie rolls
- 4 eggs
- 4 Canadian bacon slices, cooked and crisped
- 1 tablespoon white vinegar
- 1 teaspoon chives

Directions

1. Boil water with vinegar and create a whirlpool in it with a wooden spoon.
2. Break an egg in a cup and place in the boiling water for about 3 minutes.
3. Repeat with rest of the eggs and dish out onto a platter.
4. Place oopsie rolls on the plates and top with bacon slices.
5. Put the poached eggs onto bacon slices and garnish with chives to serve.

Nutrition:
Calories   190
Total Fat 13.5g
Saturated Fat 5.8g
Cholesterol 275mg
Sodium 587mg
Total Carbohydrate 1.5g
Dietary Fiber 0g
Total Sugars 0.6g
Protein 15.3g

21 Days Meal Plan

Day	Breakfast	Lunch	Dinner
1	Shrimp Skillet	Curried Chicken wrap	Shrimp Cocktail
2	Coconut Yogurt with Chia Seeds	Open-Faced Garden Tuna Sandwich	Quinoa and Scallops Salad
3	Chia Pudding	Baked Macaroni	Squid and Shrimp Salad
4	Egg Fat Bombs	Zucchini Pad Thai	Parsley Seafood Cocktail
5	Morning "Grits"	Easy Roasted Salmon	Shrimp and Onion Ginger Dressing
6	Scotch Eggs	Shrimp with Pasta, Artichoke, and Spinach	Fruit Shrimp Soup
7	Bacon Sandwich	Pistachio Crusted Halibut with Spicy Yogurt	Mussels and Chickpea Soup
8	Noatmeal	Paella with Chicken, Leeks, and Tarragon	Fish Stew
9	Breakfast Bake with Meat	Roasted Brussels Sprouts, Chicken, and Potatoes	Shrimp and Broccoli Soup
10	Breakfast Bagel	Shepherd's Pie	Coconut Turkey Mix
11	Egg and Vegetable Hash	Salmon and Edamame Cakes	Lime Shrimp and Kale
12	Cowboy Skillet	Flat Bread Pizza	Parsley Cod Mix
13	Feta Quiche	Spinach Salad with Walnuts and Strawberry	Salmon and Cabbage Mix
14	Bacon Pancakes	Chicken Vegetable Soup	Decent Beef and Onion Stew
15	Waffles	Avocado Sandwich with Lemon and Cilantro	Clean Parsley and Chicken Breast
16	Rolled Omelette with Mushrooms	Tofu and Mushroom Burger	Zucchini Beef Sauté with Coriander Greens
17	Quiche Lorraine	Cobb Salad	Hearty Lemon and Pepper Chicken
18	Breakfast Zucchini Bread	Veggie Sushi	Walnuts and Asparagus Delight
19	Granola	Curried Chicken wrap	Healthy Carrot Chips
20	Cheddar Souffle	Open-Faced Garden Tuna Sandwich	Beef Soup
21	Mediterranean Omelette	Baked Macaroni	Shrimp Cocktail

Conclusion

The Dash Diet is designed to help ladies lose weight and stay healthy. There are many useful tips and easy recipes in this cookbook that can help you better understand the Dash Diet and make healthy food choices.

Even if you aren't following the Dash Diet, this cookbook can help you need a well-made, delicious meal. At Dash Diet, we understand that our products' quality is just as important as the quality of our products. That is why Dash Diet uses hardened steel components for its ratchets.

Our ratchets are made with hardened steel that is hand-polished and handcrafted by experts in the USA. This ensures a long life for your new tool. Each part is made with precision to ensure a strong bond between the ratchet tool's male and female heads. Most people don't use their kitchen knives for cooking. Most people don't know that you should always wash them after cutting something, primarily if you've used a grinder on them.

The Dash Diet Cookbook will have you hacking out your cutlery in no time so you can finally become a healthier human being! It's all about being healthy and learning to enjoy the foods you eat again. We have concluded that Dash Diet Cookbook is an excellent way of losing weight and following a healthy, balanced diet. Our editors and team are hard at work putting together another fantastic Dash Diet cookbook that will be available in December. Keep checking back for exclusive Dash Diet products that will be sold only at Dash Diet! The Dash Diet Cookbook is a collection of simple recipes that are easy to prepare and incredibly tasty. Many different styles of cooking are featured, so you can find something that works for you. The Dash Diet Cookbook is perfect for anyone who wants to eat better and feel great while saving money and time.

If you're ready to get started, the Dash Diet Cookbook is here to help. There's something for everyone in this book, from breakfast items like oatmeal and French toast to dinner side dishes like zucchini noodles and ranch dressing. Feel great about what you eat with the Dash Diet Cookbook!

This guide is your guide to the Dash Diet Cookbook. If you have been following the diet for any amount of time, you will appreciate the information in this guide. Take advantage of the resources that were provided in this guide to ensure that you succeed on a diet.

It appears that some people have expressed concern about the lack of a portion specified in the diet. While there are no food requirements listed in the diet, it does teach you how to make healthy meals and snacks from the foods listed in the recipes. After learning how to cook Dash recipes, anyone can create a healthy and delicious meal with the right ingredients. The Dash Diet Cookbook teaches you how to plan, so you don't have to stress over making your meals before you get home from work.

INDEX

D

E

M

N

O

P

Q

V

W

Z

CPSIA information can be obtained
at www.ICGtesting.com
Printed in the USA
LVHW060356260621
691218LV00007B/705